Yearning and Refusal

YEARNING AND REFUSAL

An Ethnography of Female Fertility Management in Niamey, Niger

Hadiza Moussa

Edited by Alice J. Kang and Barbara M. Cooper

Translated by Natalie Kammerer

Preface by Jean-Pierre Olivier de Sardan

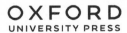
OXFORD
UNIVERSITY PRESS

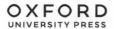

OXFORD
UNIVERSITY PRESS

Oxford University Press is a department of the University of Oxford. It furthers
the University's objective of excellence in research, scholarship, and education
by publishing worldwide. Oxford is a registered trade mark of Oxford University
Press in the UK and certain other countries.

Published in the United States of America by Oxford University Press
198 Madison Avenue, New York, NY 10016, United States of America.

Library of Congress Cataloging-in-Publication Data
Names: Moussa, Hadiza, author. | Kang, Alice J., 1978– editor. |
Cooper, Barbara MacGowan editor.
Title: Yearning and refusal : an ethnography of female fertility management
in Niamey, Niger / Hadiza Moussa ; edited by Alice J. Kang and Barbara M. Cooper ;
translated by Natalie Kammerer ; preface by Jean-Pierre Olivier de Sardan.
Other titles: Entre absence et refus d'enfant. English
Description: New York : Oxford University Press, [2023] |
Includes bibliographical references and index.
Identifiers: LCCN 2022044665 (print) | LCCN 2022044666 (ebook) |
ISBN 9780197662113 (paperback) | ISBN 9780197662137 (epub) | ISBN 9780197662144
Subjects: MESH: Infertility, Female—therapy | Anthropology, Cultural |
Health Knowledge, Attitudes, Practice | Niger | Case Reports
Classification: LCC RG201 (print) | LCC RG201 (ebook) | NLM WP 570 |
DDC 618.1/78—dc23/eng/20230103
LC record available at https://lccn.loc.gov/2022044665
LC ebook record available at https://lccn.loc.gov/2022044666

DOI: 10.1093/oso/9780197662113.001.0001

Printed by Integrated Books International, United States of America

This volume is an abridged and edited translation of *Entre absence et refus d'enfant. Socio-
anthropologie de la gestion de la fécondité féminine à Niamey, Niger*, by Hadiza Moussa, published in
French by coédition L'Harmattan/La Sahélienne, copyright: La Sahélienne, 2012.

I dedicate this book to

my father, who was unexpectedly taken away from us;

my beloved daughter Gaïcha, otherwise affectionately known as Tamarwalt;

my dear grandmother Hadjé Derey, to whom I owe everything.

CONTENTS

LIST OF FIGURES AND TABLES

EDITORS' INTRODUCTION

Alice J. Kang and Barbara M. Cooper

Yearning and Refusal explores the practical and emotional realities of women's reproductive health in a Muslim majority country, the Republic of Niger. The book examines two dimensions of reproductive health that are crucial to improving the well-being of women in West Africa and elsewhere. Both, paradoxically, concern *failures* to produce children. The author, Hadiza Moussa, reveals the lived experience of women who are struggling with infertility, on the one hand, and of women who refuse to become or to remain pregnant, on the other. Her empirical research draws attention to phenomena societal leaders, politicians, and public health specialists have tended to evade or neglect. Almost no work uniting these issues— infertility and contraception—under a common theoretical framework has been written. Yet infertility and contraception are the poles that define the reproductive experiences of many women.

Focusing her research in Niamey, the capital city of Niger, Moussa sets out the existential experience of failed fertility; its physical, emotional, and social implications; and how it undermines women's standing within their marriages, households, and society as a whole. Drawing upon interviews, participant observation, and her intimate knowledge of Nigerien society, she depicts the stark realities that women face, to lay bare the emotional and social consequences of the failure to address effectively either the problem of infertility or the problem of unwanted pregnancies. By seeking out contraception and illicit abortions, women in Niamey refuse to produce children willy-nilly, despite the pressures of their husbands, in-laws, and society as a whole. Moussa shows that women are far from passive with regard to their fertility and have long sought ways to control it. Yet the strategies available to them do not fundamentally challenge or alter dominant sexual and reproductive norms.

Niger's population growth rate, the highest in the world, is a near obsession among news outlets, scientists, and international organizations in the West. "Why Have Four Children when You Could Have Seven? Family Planning in Niger" asks one headline from the British newspaper *The Guardian* (Filipovic 2017). "Niger Has the World's Highest Birth Rate—And That May Be a Recipe for Unrest," reads the title of a think piece in *The Conversation* (May 2019). An article in *Nature* that advocates for family planning states, "Avert Catastrophe Now in Africa's Sahel" (Graves et al. 2019). Western policymakers generally see Niger's fertility rate as an environmental and security threat and a hindrance to the realization of women's empowerment—and they are not entirely wrong (Graves, Moumouni, and Potts 2021). These concerns undergird the more than $370 million spent by the European Union, Canada, the United States, the United Nations, the World Bank, and other agencies on population policy and reproductive health in Niger between 2002 and 2018 (Organisation for Economic Co-operation and Development 2020).

THE PROBLEM OF INFERTILITY

Married women in Niger do appear to have begun to respond in modest ways to family planning initiatives. Women over the past three decades have initiated childbearing slightly later and space births slightly further apart than previously. This has not yet dramatically altered the overall numbers of children they bear; this new spacing results in what demographers refer to as "fertility compression" rather than fertility reduction (Spoorenberg and Maga 2018). However, in the focus on *fertility reduction*, policymakers in the West have tended to overlook the fact that Niger, like many other countries in Africa, has high rates of *infertility*. Some researchers have estimated that 9% of couples worldwide experience infertility (Boivin et al. 2007; Ombelet et al. 2008). In an incidence/exposure study drawing upon Demographic and Health Survey data on 14 countries in Africa, infertility—defined as the inability to conceive after an initial pregnancy—affected more than one in four women (Rutstein and Shah 2004).

It is notoriously hard to measure infertility because definitions vary and data collection is not uniform. One contemporary definition would be the failure of a woman in a couple to give birth within two years of regular unprotected sex (Akhondi et al. 2019). Many couples and their families in Niger and elsewhere become impatient well before two years have passed— the perception of infertility is in many ways more socially relevant than the medical or demographic determination. In any case, in the face of population growth and poverty, however, Niger's infertility rate is not a prominent political or policy concern (Cooper 2013). Jade Sasser points out that Western preoccupations with African women's fertility—rather than infertility—are unlikely to go away as private donors, scientists, and environmental activists target African women's reproduction as a driver of global climate change (2018).

One of the major contributions of Hadiza Moussa's work is to show that women in Niger who do not produce children at the appropriate moment—and quickly enough—experience that failure as a crisis of personhood. Involuntary childlessness can strike both men and women, and it can affect those who have never conceived, those who have already given birth, and those whose pregnancies repeatedly miscarry. Picking up on a major theme in the research of anthropologists and sociologists studying West Africa (e.g., the work of Yannick Jaffré), Moussa pays attention to the actual social and emotional experiences of women seeking treatment for their fertility issues. Hadiza Moussa's sensitive study of the emotional life of subfertile individuals contributes to a growing call to attend not simply to the physiological problem of infertility but also to the urgent emotional, social, and psychological dimensions of the quest to manage one's fertility (Armah et al. 2021; Duffy et al. 2020).

The urgent problem of infertility in Africa was brought to light in Anne Retel-Laurentin's groundbreaking *Infécondité en Afrique noire*, published in 1974. Despite its significance, the topic languished for many years as scholars focused instead on genital cutting, human immunodeficiency virus/AIDS, and contraceptive prevalence rates. Important research on infertility focusing upon assisted reproductive technologies (ARTs) across the globe was launched in the 1990s by Marcia Inhorn (1994; Inhorn and van Balen 2002) and Doris Bonnet and Veronique Duchesne (2016). Many excellent monographs in English take up fertility and infertility: in Egypt (Inhorn 1994), Cameroon (Feldman-Savelsberg 1999; Johnson-Hanks 2006), Nigeria (Renne 1996), and Mali (Sassens 2001).

Yet it is the *absence* of opportunities to seek out ARTs that constitutes the lived reality of most subfertile women in Africa, a reality that deserves its own attention. Researchers in English-speaking countries in Africa (Ghana, Nigeria, and South Africa) find that women with fertility issues are more likely to experience stress, depression, anxiety, and intimate partner violence (Ameh et al. 2007; Donkor and Sandall 2007; Naab, Brown, and Heidrich 2013; Upkong and Orji 2007; Boerma and Mgalla 2001). Infertility rates are highest in poorer countries with very little access to ARTs and where the implications of sterility fall heavily upon women (Inhorn and

Patrizio 2015). There has been so little access to ARTs on the continent (with the exception of South Africa, Ghana, Nigeria, and Egypt) that the development of clinics, as well as research on the appropriation of ARTs, is still in its infancy. When interviewing fertility experts in Africa in 2009, Viola Horbst found that they insisted that "you cannot do IVF in Africa as in Europe" (2016: 108).

Seeking to historicize such reproductive issues in a former French colony, Barbara Cooper studied the history of childbirth in Niger to illuminate the institutional, social, religious, and emotional origins of the high fertility and infertility rates in the Sahel (2019). She found Hadiza Moussa's rich ethnography to be one of the very few full-length monographs on infertility in Africa published in French. Moussa's book is therefore a particularly welcome contribution to work on infertility in Africa and deserves to be well known among scholars working in English.

UNWELCOME CHILDBEARING

In the focus upon contraceptive prevalence rates in discussions of Niger's high population growth rate, another key problem has been neglected. A strong pro-natal sentiment prevents women from going to public health clinics for contraception. The stigma attached to contraceptive use is high. Inevitably, some women fall pregnant at times that are not ideal for them. Such women are often married and want to "rest" or space their births more effectively. Others feel that they or their husbands simply don't have the resources to support another child at that time. In Niger, women's efforts to control the timing of pregnancy have often been framed in the context of a highly politicized contest between a purportedly imported Western feminism and a purportedly purified Islam (Cooper 2019). Under these circumstances many women seek contraception of a variety of kinds in secret. In effect, in the absence of discrete access to contraception, some turn to induced abortion as a form of contraception.

With the exceptions of South Africa (Klausen 2015), Zambia (Haaland et al. 2019), Tunisia (Hajri et al. 2015), Cape Verde, Mozambique and recently Benin (Peltier 2022) abortion is anathema throughout most of the continent. Despite the fatal outcomes and adverse sequelae of the induced abortions that inevitably result, the taboo on abortion has slowed the pace of research and the pursuit of solutions to the problem of unsafe abortions. Women's experiences with abortion and contraception have gained attention more recently, often from scholars based on the continent (e.g., Diarra et al. 2017; Mogobe 2005; Okonofua 1999; Okafor, Joe-Ikechebelu, and

Ikechebelu 2017; Storeng and Ouattara 2014; Ouédraogo 2015; Naab and Heidrich 2014; Rossier et al. 2006). Both surgical and medication-induced abortions are illegal in Niger. Nevertheless, as Hadiza Moussa reveals, women make use of a variety of "grandmother's" recipes, toxic substances rumored to have the desired effect, and the covert assistance of medically trained individuals to terminate pregnancies.

Such contraceptive abortions are visible in government statistics only when something goes wrong. That is, an abortion becomes "data" when a woman who seeks post-abortion care in a medical facility is reported to the police by a healthcare provider. A sympathetic nurse might choose to handle such a case discreetly as a "spontaneous abortion" or miscarriage, but there is little sympathy for women who have had an abortion in general. The medical treatment of women seeking post-abortion care, as Siri Suh (2021) has shown for Senegal, is hindered by a general distaste for the equipment and techniques associated with inducing abortion. This danger does not deter women in Africa from seeking out clandestine abortions or some trained specialists from performing them (Koster 2003). Safe, medically supervised abortions, because they are illegal, pass under the radar (Diarra et al. 2017). By interviewing women at some remove from the medical setting, Hadiza Moussa provides rare insight into what they think about induced abortions, how they seek them out, and why.

THEORETICAL ORIENTATIONS AND ABSENCES

Moussa's doctoral training at the École des Hautes Études en Sciences Sociales (EHESS) and the studies she conducted as a researcher at the Laboratoire d'Études et de Recherches sur les Dynamiques Sociales et le Développement Local (LASDEL, Laboratory for the Study and Research of Social Dynamics and Local Development) undoubtedly informed her approach to studying infertility and contraception. In addition, Moussa had several lodestars that oriented her thinking. Intriguingly, she found in the social history of early modern France insights that bring contemporary reproductive life in Niger closer than one might have expected to life in pre-industrial Europe. The idea of studying struggles to become pregnant and struggles to avoid giving birth in a single work emerged in part from that comparative reading, in particular the work of Jacques Gélis. It was his 1984 book *L'arbre et le fruit* that inspired her to do a research project bringing together infertility and efforts at avoiding fertility. The goal in this comparative frame was not to suggest that Niger is in a throwback to an earlier time in Europe but rather to note the ways that particular family structures give rise to patterned gender dynamics.

Moussa took considerable inspiration from the works of the major French anthropologist and feminist thinker Françoise Héritier in her analysis of the gender dynamics driving marriage and sexuality. Héritier studied at length the implications of the "valence differentielle des sexes" or the inequality between men and women and the nature of masculine domination as derived from the construction of bodily difference (1981, 50). In the spirit of Claude Lévi-Strauss, she argued that this fundamental difference is encountered over and over in the binary oppositions structuring every social field, in effect rendering masculine domination seemingly natural. Héritier's insight that masculine power rests fundamentally on the control of women's bodies and their reproductive capacity clearly informs Moussa's work. Moussa also consulted the work of a host of other women anthropologists writing in French on issues related to fertility, infertility, contraception, and abortion for comparative material to buttress her efforts to generalize about the phenomena she describes (Armelle Andro, Véronique Hertrich, Sylvie Fainzang, Nicole Echard, and Suzanne Lallemand). She was evidently unaware of the works published in English by Marcia Inhorn, Caroline Bledsoe, Pamela Feldman-Savelsberg, Jennifer Johnson-Hanks, and Saskia Sassens.

Moussa did have access to the work of sociologist Erving Goffman in translation. His reflections on the nature of stigma were crucial to her understanding of infertility and to her approach to studying emotion. She thought deeply about how emotion emerged out of interactions between individuals and how important shame and "saving face" are to the formation of a sense of self in the context of reproduction. An approach through what she refers to often as "semiology" was helpful in her eventual understanding of the psychological patterns and processes she learned about from her informants. The words and expressions she explores have meaning within broader sets of relationships and particularly in light of the contrasts they imply and the associations they produce. While her approach to her ethnographic evidence is reflexive and she is interested centrally in symbolic interaction, her use of semiotics is what Peter Manning would characterize as "loose" (2011, 15). Although she makes close analysis of discourse and metaphoric speech, she doesn't deploy the vocabulary associated with Saussurean semiotics. For example, she is attentive to the broad semantic fields of particular words, such as *haawi* (roughly "shame"); but she does not engage in the analysis of signs or codes for the purpose of engaging directly with post-structuralism.

Moussa conducted her study in the ethnically and socially diverse city of Niamey, where in her interviews she moved easily between Zarma and Hausa. The choice to conduct the study in Niamey had implications for some of her thinking. Had she done her research in the Hausa region of Maradi, she might have found herself reflecting more deeply upon *bori* spirit possession practices, for example, which continue to have tremendous social, spiritual, and therapeutic significance. There is a great deal of literature on the significance of *bori*, *holey*, *zar*, and other spirit possession cults in Africa for creating spaces for the hermeneutics and treatment of sexual and reproductive concerns (Lewis et al. 1991; Boddy 1989; Masquelier 2001; Gaudio 2009). Indeed, the relationship between the spirit and the medium is often thought of as a marriage. Yet Moussa devotes a scant handful of paragraphs to the social milieu of those drawn to *bori* and *holey*. Perhaps she felt that spirit possession has been overemphasized by outsiders, or perhaps she feared that it might not be seen as a "serious" topic for a dissertation. The reticence of the healers she approached suggests they did not trust her, nor she them, making it less likely that they would open the way to her to become more familiar with that milieu.

The choice not to focus upon possession comes at considerable cost—in her effort to show the significance of childbearing for women's full entry into womanhood, she effectively reinscribes the very binary she critiques. What of the "women" who find a home in *bori*, where their *incapacity* to give birth is transmuted into a *capacity* to engage with the spiritual realm, to heal others, and to attend to the psychic scars generated by heteronormative marriage? What of the "men" whose gender-non-conforming dress, effeminate speech, pleasure in sex with other men, and immersion in a non-homosocial environment fly in the face of the expectations of procreative masculinity? Moussa's approach leaves little room for any third-space sexuality. It also leaves unexplored the crucial question of whether gender-binary non-conforming individuals negotiate socially male or female self-presentation through reproduction. Precisely because, as Rudy Gaudio (2018, 361) has observed, "queer Africans' lives and struggles are embedded in and connected to broader sociopolitical phenomena that affect all Africans" they might have brought fresh insight into the meanings and experiences of marriage and infertility in Niger.

Given that we two editors also struggle with the ways that heteronormativity frames our research questions and fieldwork in Niger, it would be unfair of us to be too critical of her on that front! Her research was very much bound up in the preoccupations of her "subjects." This was the world she herself navigated as a woman academic, a wife, and a researcher—it was difficult enough to talk about sexuality in any form, as she notes in her own introductory chapter. No single study can accomplish everything. *Yearning and Refusal*, as we have translated the title of her book, offers rich ethnographic observations and extraordinary interview material on the lived experiences of infertile sexuality. The juxtaposition of infertility and contraception she models offers a far better grasp of the existential, emotional, and psychological dimensions of conjugal debt than we have hitherto seen. Her agile and sensitive analysis of emotion, language, and social interaction makes this a deeply rewarding book to read.

ON THE TRANSLATION PROCESS

Alice Kang first met Hadiza Moussa at LASDEL around 2007 when they were both doctoral students. Over the years the two met in Niamey to catch up and share their research with each other. Their conversations shaped Kang's research for *Bargaining for Women's Rights* (2015), for example, leading her to consider the significance of curses against women leaders more seriously. Barbara Cooper came to know Hadiza Moussa also at LASDEL after Moussa had completed her degree. Cooper was deeply grateful to Moussa for sharing her extraordinary dissertation, which became an invaluable resource as she struggled to understand reproductive concerns in contemporary Niamey while writing *Countless Blessings* (2019).

Hadiza Moussa suffered an untimely death in a car accident in 2013, not long after the publication of her book *Entre absence et refus d'enfant: Socio-anthropologie de la gestion de la fécondité féminine à Niamey, Niger* (2012). Recognizing the significance of her work, we decided to translate it to reach students, scholars, and policymakers who work primarily in English. The original French publication was a lightly revised version of the dissertation Moussa wrote for her doctorate in anthropology from EHESS in France in 2008. In 2014, we began making inquiries into the translation of Moussa's book with her husband Moussa Zangaou and dissertation advisor Jean-Pierre Olivier de Sardan. We asked Susan Cox to translate one chapter, which she did before her passing. We later commissioned Natalie Kammerer to translate most of the rest of the book. That translation was then considerably reworked and edited by the two of us to make it short enough for publication given the trend in academic presses to produce shorter books.

We had to make a number of decisions in transforming a French-language dissertation into an English-language monograph. For example, we rendered the authorial "we" as "I," and unexpectedly the manuscript became much more intimate. We sought to ensure consistency across chapters, reduce redundancy, and remove unnecessary references to secondary literature. We sometimes found that moving the concluding sentence to the beginning of each chapter to serve as a thesis statement improved the flow of her writing and made it possible to tighten the material. We combined and reordered some paragraphs to avoid repeating evidence multiple times. Some of this cutting enabled us to move material that had been relegated to footnotes into the text, where it belonged. Moussa's original ideas and ethnographic research now emerge more clearly. In other words, this is an edited and abridged translation, not a word-for-word rendition of the original into English.

Perhaps the biggest change we made was to craft a pivotal chapter between the first part of the book, on infertility, and the second, on contraception and abortion. That new Chapter 5, "Confronting the Biomedical Sphere," is a sustained discussion of the experiences of women seeking reproductive health services in government medical facilities. In the original text, this material was presented in several different places in the book. Hadiza Moussa, through her work as a researcher at LASDEL, knew a great deal about the problems women face in health clinics and hospitals (see her studies cited by Jean-Pierre Olivier de Sardan in his Preface). When brought together, Moussa's evidence provides a clear sense for why women do not always feel comfortable in health centers and why they pursue multiple therapeutic solutions even when the cost of biomedical care is manageable. The chapter also serves as a springboard for understanding why and how an illegal reproductive health economy exists.

The first part of the original book was intended to provide background for the second and third parts. In the interest of space, we combined her "general introduction" and this background material into a single introductory chapter. We included in full her description of her methodology and most of the contextual material she provided on reproductive norms. Her literature review, which demonstrates her command of different research approaches, was too long to include in its entirety. We retained the discussions of the books and ideas that she referred to again later in the text.

We decided to translate the French term *infécondité* as "infertility" rather than "sterility" to capture the spectrum of sentiments and experiences that accompany the failure to produce children as well as the latest discussions of the appropriate vocabulary to use. Reproductive health practitioners and researchers today agree that "subfertility" and "infertility" can be used interchangeably (Zegers-Hochschild et al. 2017). However, they are not the same thing as sterility, which is the biological inability to produce a live birth.

In writing African languages in Roman letters, Hadiza Moussa followed francophone conventions rather than those more familiar in English. We have retained her original orthography out of a concern to be as faithful as possible to the original interviews. We have occasionally provided notes where Moussa assumes a familiarity with a concept that is unlikely to be well known to our readers. We also use notes to reference additional literature or updated information that would be useful to the reader. Such comments are marked as an "Editor's note" to distinguish them from her own notes.

Ideally, making a translation would entail many conversations between the author and translator. Producing a posthumous translation turned out to be painful at times because we could not consult with our friend and colleague. We are nevertheless confident that this lovingly edited translation is faithful to her ideas. We are grateful to the family of Hadiza Moussa, particularly her husband Moussa Zangaou, for their support for the translation of her book into English. Jean-Pierre Olivier de Sardan facilitated contact with Moussa's publisher and graciously wrote an updated preface to this edition. Soumana Cissé, Zeinabou Hadari, and Abdoulaye Sounaye offered valuable advice and encouragement. We thank Ismaïla Samba Traoré at Editions La Sahélienne in Bamako, Mali, for granting the copyright for the English translation; Sarah Humphreville and Emma Hodgdon at Oxford University Press and Prabha Karunakaran of Newgen for shepherding this edition into the world; and Diana Witt for preparing the index.

We would like to acknowledge the financial support of the College of Arts and Sciences at the University of Nebraska-Lincoln. Summer salary enabled Alice Kang to pay for the first few stages of the project. We would also like to acknowledge with gratitude the support of Rutgers University in providing the research funds we used to pay Natalie Kammerer to complete the second half of the translation. During a cash flow crisis as we shifted from one source of funding to another, we turned to friends and colleagues for assistance through a GoFundMe page. We thank Caroline Agalheir, Ousseina Alidou, Sarah Burgess, Catherine Day, Rutu Chhatre, David Corbin, Halimatou Hima, Bonnie Huber, Hilary Hungerford, Thomas Kelley, Brandon Kendhammer, Gabriella Körling, Kristi Montooth, Lisa Mueller, Eric Schmidt, Daizaburo Shizuka, Viet Nguyen, Rebecca Popenoe, Jimmy Wang, Jacqueline Wheelwright, and Charlotte Whitney for providing a lifeline at a critical moment and for recognizing the importance of bringing Hadiza Moussa's incomparable book to an English-reading audience.

BIBLIOGRAPHY

Akhondi, Mohammad Mehdi, Fahime Ranjbar, Mahdi Shirzad, et al. 2019. Practical difficulties in estimating the prevalence of primary infertility in Iran. *International Journal of Fertility and Sterility* 13 (2): 113–117.

Ameh, Nkeiruka., T. S. Kene, S. O. Onuh, et al. 2007. Burden of domestic violence amongst infertile women attending infertility clinics in Nigeria. *Nigerian Journal of Medicine* 16 (4): 375–377.

Armah, Deborah, Annatjie van der Wath, Mariatha Yazbek, and Florence Naab. 2021. Holistic management of female infertility: a systematic review. *African Journal of Reproductive Health* 25 (2): 150–161.

Boddy, Janice. 1989. *Wombs and alien spirits: women, men, and the Zar cult in northern Sudan.* Madison: Wisconsin University Press.

Boerma, J. T., and Zaida Mgalla, eds. 2001. *Women and infertility in sub-Saharan Africa: a multi-disciplinary perspective.* Amsterdam: Royal Tropical Institute.

Boivin, Jacky, Laura Bunting, John Collins, and Karl Nygren. 2007. International estimates of infertility prevalence and treatment-seeking: potential need and demand for infertility medical care. *Human Reproduction* 22 (6): 1506–1512.

Bonnet, Doris, and Véronique Duchesne, eds. 2016. *Procréation médicale et mondialisation: expériences africaines.* Paris: L'Harmattan.

Cooper, Barbara M. 2013. De quoi la crise démographique au Sahel est-elle le nom? *Politique Africaine* 2 (130): 69–88.

Cooper, Barbara M. 2019. *Countless blessings: a history of childbirth and reproduction in the Sahel.* Bloomington: Indiana University Press.

Diarra, Aïssa, et al. 2017. Les interruptions volontaires de grossesse au Niger. *Etudes et travaux du LASDEL* 128: 1–88.

Donkor, Ernestina S., and Jane Sandall. 2007. The impact of perceived stigma and mediating social factors on infertility-related stress among women seeking infertility treatment in southern Ghana. *Social Science and Medicine* 65 (8): 1683–1694.

Duffy, James M. N., G. David Adamnson, E. Benson, et al. 2020. Top 10 priorities for future infertility research: an international consensus development study. *Human Reproduction* 35 (12): 2715–2724.

Feldman-Savelsberg, Pamela. 1999. *Plundered kitchens, empty wombs: threatened reproduction and identity in the Cameroon grassfields.* Ann Arbor: University of Michigan Press.

Filipovic, Jill. 2017. Why have four children when you could have seven? Family planning in Niger. *The Guardian*, March 15.

Gaudio, Rudolf. 2009. *Allah made us: sexual outlaws in an Islamic African city.* Malden, MA: Wiley-Blackwell.

Gaudio, Rudolf. 2018. Queer as kin: reflections on the twentieth anniversary of *Boy-Wives and Female Husbands: studies in African Homosexualities. Canadian Journal of African Studies* 52 (3): 359–361.

Gélis, Jacques. 1984. *L'arbre et le fruit : la naissance dans l'Occident moderne, XVIe-XIXe siècle.* Paris: Fayard.

Graves, Alisha, Nouhou Abdoul Moumouni, and Malcolm Potts. 2021. Demography and health in the context of climate change. In *The Oxford handbook of the African Sahel*, ed. Leonardo Villalon, 249–267. Oxford: Oxford University Press.

Graves, Alisha, Lorenzo Rosa, Abdoul Moumouni Nouhou, et al. 2019. Avert catastrophe now in Africa's Sahel. *Nature,* November 13.

Haaland, Marte E. S., Haldis Haukanes, Joseph Mumba Zulu, et al. 2019. Shaping the abortion policy: competing discourses on the Zambian Termination of Pregnancy Act. *International Journal of Equity Health* 18: 20. https://doi.org/10.1186/s12939-018-0908-8

Hajri, Selma, Sarah Raifman, Caitlin Gerdts, et al. 2015. "This is real misery": experiences of women denied legal abortion in Tunisia. *PLoS One* 10 (12): e0145338.

Héritier, Françoise. 1981. *L'exercice de la parenté.* Paris: Gallimard-Le-Seuil.

Hörbst, Viola. 2016. "You cannot do IVF in Africa as in Europe": the making of IVF in Mali and Uganda. *Reproductive Biomedicine & Society Online* 2: 108–115.

Inhorn, Marcia. 1994. *Quest for conception: gender, infertility, and Egyptian medical traditions.* Philadelphia: University of Pennsylvania Press.

Inhorn, Marcia C., and Pasquale Patrizio. 2015. Infertility around the globe: new thinking on gender, reproductive technologies, and global movements in the 21st century. *Human Reproduction Update* 21 (4): 411–426.

Inhorn, Marcia C., and Frank van Balen, eds. 2002. *Infertility around the globe: new thinking on childlessness, gender, and reproductive technologies.* Berkeley: University of California Press.

Johnson-Hanks, Jennifer. 2006. *Uncertain honor: modern motherhood in an African crisis.* Chicago: University of Chicago Press.

Kang, Alice. 2015. *Bargaining for women's rights: activism in an aspiring Muslim democracy.* Minneapolis: University of Minnesota Press.

Klausen, Susanne. 2015. *Abortion under apartheid: nationalism, sexuality and women's reproductive rights in South Africa.* New York: Oxford University Press.

Koster, Winny. 2003. *Secret strategies: women and abortion in Yoruba society, Nigeria.* Amsterdam: Aksant.

Lewis, I. M., et al. 1991. *Women's medicine: the Zar-bori cult in Africa and beyond.* Edinburgh: Edinburgh University Press for the International African Institute.

Manning, Peter K. 2011. Semiotics, semantics and ethnography. In *Handbook of ethnography,* eds. Paul Atkinson et al., 145–159. Newbury Park: SAGE Research Methods. https://doi.org/10.4135/9781848608337

Masquelier, Adeline. 2001. *Prayer has spoiled everything: possession, power, and identity in an Islamic town of Niger.* Durham, NC: Duke University Press.

May, John F. 2019. Niger has the world's highest birth rate—and that may be a recipe for unrest. *The Conversation,* March 21. https://theconversation.com/niger-has-the-worlds-highest-birth-rate-and-that-may-be-a-recipe-for-unrest-108654

Mogobe, Dintle K. 2005. Denying and preserving self: Batswana women's experiences of infertility. *African Journal of Reproductive Health* 9 (2): 26–37.

Moussa, Hadiza. 2012. *Entre absence et refus d'enfant: Socio-anthropologie de la gestion de la fécondité féminine à Niamey, Niger.* Paris: L'Harmattan.

Naab, Florence, Roger Brown, and Susan Heidrich. 2013. Psychosocial health of infertile Ghanaian women and their infertility beliefs. *Journal of Nursing Scholarship* 45 (2): 132–140.

Naab, Florence, and Susan Heidrich. 2014. Common sense understanding of infertility among Ghanaian women with infertility. *Journal of Infertility and Reproductive Biology* 2 (1): 11–22.

Okafor, Nneka I., Ngozi N. Joe-Ikechebelu, and Joseph I. Ikechebelu. 2017. Perceptions of infertility and in vitro fertilization treatment among married couples in Anambra state, Nigeria. *African Journal of Reproductive Health* 21 (4): 55–66.

Okonofua, Friday. 1999. Infertility and women's reproductive health. *African Journal of Reproductive Health* 3 (1): 7–12.

Ombelet, Willem, Ian Cooke, Silke Dyer, et al. 2008. Infertility and the provision of infertility medical services in developing countries. *Human Reproduction Update* 14 (6): 605–621.

Organisation for Economic Co-operation and Development. 2020. Query wizard for international development statistics. Accessed December 16, 2020. https://stats.oecd.org/qwids/.

Ouédraogo, Ramatou. 2015. Les méthodes contraceptives rendent stérile. In *Des idées reçues en santé mondiale*, eds. Valery Ridde and Fatoumata Ouattara, 73–77. Montréal: Presses de l'Université de Montréal.

Renne, Elisha P. 1996. Perceptions of population policy, development, and family planning programs in northern Nigeria. *Studies in Family Planning* 27 (3): 127–136.

Retel-Laurentin, Anne. 1974. *Infécondité en Afrique noire: maladies et conséquences sociales*. Paris: Masson et Cie.

Rossier C, G. Guiella, A. Ouédraogo, and B. Thiéba. 2006. Estimating clandestine abortion with the confidants method—results from Ouagadougou, Burkina Faso. *Social Science & Medicine* 62 (1): 254–266.

Rutstein, Shea O., and Iqbal H. Shah. 2004. *Infecundity, infertility, and childlessness in developing countries*. DHS Comparative Reports no. 9. Calverton, MD: ORC Macros and the World Health Organization.

Sassens, Saskia. 2001. *Mediating means and fate: a socio-political analysis of fertility and demographic change in Bamako, Mali*. Leiden: Brill.

Sasser, Jade. 2018. *On infertile ground: population control and women's rights in the era of climate change*. New York: NYU Press.

Spoorenberg, Thomas, and Hamidou Issaka Maga. 2018. Fertility compression in Niger: a study of fertility change by parity (1977–2011). *Demographic Research* 39 (24): 685–700.

Storeng, Katerini T. and Fatoumata Ouattara. 2014. The politics of unsafe abortion in Burkina Faso: the interface of local norms and global public health practice. *Global Public Health* 9 (8): 946–959.

Suh, Siri. 2021. *Dying to count: post-abortion care and global reproductive health politics in Senegal*. New Brunswick: Rutgers University Press.

Upkong, Dominic, and Eo Orji. 2007. Mental health of infertile women in Nigeria. *Turkish Journal of Psychiatry* 17 (4): 259–265.

Zegers-Hochschild, Fernando, G. David Adamson, Silke Dyer, et al. 2017. The international glossary on infertility and fertility care. *Human Reproduction* 32 (9): 1786–1801.

PREFACE FOR THE ENGLISH TRANSLATION

Jean-Pierre Olivier de Sardan

There are two statistics that usually dominate the landscape of mother-hood in Niger: the fertility rate and the maternal mortality rate. These are, respectively, 7.2 births per woman (2016) and 535 deaths per 100,000 births (2014), making Niger's fertility rate one of the highest in the world and placing it among the 15 countries where women are most likely to die in childbirth. These data define "structural contexts": they establish both a worrisome demographic pressure (considering the fragility of food re-sources and the vulnerability of households) and a major public health issue.

Various public policies use these statistics as a basis for their objectives, arguments, and operations. For example, Western countries, worried about what is sometimes called the "demographic bomb" in the Sahel and its possible consequences for migration to Europe or for the advance-ment of Islamic terrorism, have increased pressures and incentives for the African countries concerned, particularly Niger, to promote birth spacing, family planning, and the dissemination of contraceptive techniques. Furthermore, a great many northern non-governmental organizations in-clude such services in their programs. Maternal mortality is a priority for global public health, and the protocols promoted by international organi-zations are reaching Nigerien health facilities.

But behind these figures, behind the array of indicators used by public policy, behind structural contexts, "pragmatic contexts" (i.e., the contexts experienced, perceived, and practiced by the actors concerned) are some-what different. Social, family, and biographical constraints weigh on women's lived experience, as illustrated through specific cases and life stories. Joy, of course, but also much suffering are discernable just beneath the surface of these blunt, dry statistics: Halima gave birth to 10 children, of whom only four are still alive; Ramatou had three stillborn children and died during her fourth delivery.

What's more, other facets of women's reproductive experience are invisible in these statistics and ignored by health policymakers. There hides another tragedy. The pain of sterility. The pain of induced abortion. Little is said about these pains—they are hidden, shameful, and no figures are available to aggregate and reveal them. If doctors and nurses know them well and deal with them in the silence of their offices, the world of decision-makers and public health officials—in Niger but also more generally within the context of "global health"—turns its head and looks away. Because in the face of high population growth and massive poverty, the sterility experienced by some women is not a political issue, and the fight against sterility seems to be only a luxury of wealthy countries. Induced abortion, despite its frequently fatal outcomes and its various adverse sequelae, remains a taboo subject for religious and moral reasons, which ultimately emerge at the political level against a backdrop of hypocrisy and cowardice.

The greatest merit of Hadiza Moussa's work is that it lifts the veil, examining through empirical research what social leaders, politicians, and public health specialists ignore, neglect, or dare not discuss, in particular female sterility, on the one hand, and induced abortion, on the other. Indeed, though she addresses more generally the management of female fertility, including the regulation of births and what is still often called "family planning," female sterility is at the heart of her inquiries and analyses. This is a subject largely ignored in research on Africa (with the exception of Cooper 2013).

Female sterility is, first and foremost, an individual tragedy if a woman's desire for a child cannot be realized. But in Niger, as in many other African countries, it also occasions a social stigma that directly influences a woman's status. A wife can only reach full social realization by becoming a mother. This "pro-natalist" ideology permeates all of society. And woe to the woman who cannot conceive, unable to provide offspring to her husband. Through the many interviews she conducted with talent and rigor, Hadiza Moussa reveals the thousand and one facets of the ostracism suffered by a sterile woman: repudiation, contempt, suspicion, rumors, polygamy, etc. A central element of the story told in these pages is that the social disapproval these women experience is, paradoxically, orchestrated more by other women (mothers, sisters, friends, co-wives) than by men. Pro-natalism is certainly also reproduced by men, but in the case of childless couples, some men might feel "obligated" to take a second wife against their will under pressure from their families. It should also not be forgotten that, if a woman is not pregnant after one or two years of marriage, the husband is most often exonerated, at least initially, of any responsibility: infertility is first imputed to the woman by those around her.

But it is certainly the more general context that must be considered, as Hadiza Moussa reminds us throughout her book. Niger is a society strongly dominated by men, at least as far as the public sphere and social values are concerned. Of course, women have counter-powers, especially in the domestic sphere, and implement countless strategies of cunning, resistance, and circumvention—they are far from merely passive victims of male power. But it is nevertheless true that women are marginalized in political life (and often reduced to the role of child-bearer or provider of sexual services) as a result of male domination.

Islam, at least as it is interpreted and taught by most Nigerien clerics and exegetes (marabouts, ulama, imams, and sheikhs of various traditions or orders), plays an important role in this matter, providing a strong legitimation for this female "inferiority." The dramatic rise of Salafist-style fundamentalism over the past two decades has also worsened the situation of women. Other interpretations of the Qur'an are of course possible, but in Niger these remain uncommon and are rarely discussed.

It is on the subject of polygamy that social and Islamic values merge most closely, and this phenomenon arguably exerts the most negative effects on the status of women. Polygamy introduces jealousy and competition within the home and domestic life and is most often a powerful inducer or accelerator of rivalry between women (and their children). The Songhay-Zarma term *baabize-tarey*, which refers to relationships between children of the same father but not of the same mother, is commonly used to connote jealousy, competition, and rivalry (Olivier de Sardan 2017). It should therefore come as no surprise that the pain caused by infertility is intimately linked to polygamy—in a polygamous household, a sterile wife is in a bad position in front of her co-wives and becomes an ideal target for their insults; in a monogamous household, infertility is often the main argument for polygamy.

But we must also do justice to the pages where Hadiza Moussa moves away from the issue of involuntary infertility to focus upon what might at first appear as its antithesis: the voluntary regulation of births. What she calls "infertile sexuality" covers these two opposing ends of the spectrum. In addition to women who want a child but cannot give birth, there are indeed those who can but do not want to (at least at a given moment). This appears to be in line with donor policies, which focus on promoting birth control to reduce population growth. But Hadiza Moussa manages to show us another angle, from the perspective of the women concerned. She illustrates that the "desire not to have children" is much more prevalent among Nigerien women than might be thought. But this desire is generally temporary (a fact that family planning policies seem to ignore) and linked to four specific life stages: before marriage, during breastfeeding, as a result of marital difficulty, and when one is "tired" of having had many children. But this "desire not to have children" is confronted with many obstacles that prevent its realization: beliefs in the effectiveness of "local prevention methods" (based on magico-religious practices), innumerable difficulties of access to family planning services, taboos around premarital sex, demands from husbands, preaching by ulamas and marabouts, etc. Not to mention, here too, the effects of polygamy! Even in the opinion of many health professionals (unfortunately no figures are available), the high frequency of induced abortions, which are sometimes used as a kind of "contraceptive technique" (especially by young girls), is a significant indication both of this "desire not to have children" and of the enormous challenges women face in Niger (Diarra 2017) and in neighboring countries (Ouédraogo 2015; Sambieni and Paul 2015; Ouédraogo and Guillaume 2017).

Reading Hadiza Moussa's book, originally published in French in 2012, should leave no one indifferent. Not only does it address with courage and rigor subjects that are central to daily life, to the couple, to the family, to sexuality, yet which remain little discussed by African researchers, but it also examines them through a qualitative anthropological approach drawing heavily on interviews, observations, case studies, and documentary sources. In other words, Hadiza Moussa was true to one of the major objectives of LASDEL, our shared research institute (www.lasdel. net): fueling necessary public debate through serious empirical social science research.

Her other works take up different questions and focus on other themes, all of which exhibit the same qualities and meet the same objective. She carried out in-depth research on the place of women in the political life of one Nigerien village investigated over several years (Moussa 2005, 2007, 2011), on the daily functioning of a health facility (Moussa 2003a), on a local political arena in the far east of the country (Moussa 2003b), and on the sexual health of adolescents (Moussa and Elhadji Dagobi 2015). In each she sought to focus on the condition and experiences of women but also to describe the "real" world, often far removed from the official world, and to analyze the daily behavior of actors, much closer to informal "practical norms" (Olivier de Sardan 2015) than to requirements, rules, and procedures issued by public authorities and development institutions.

But Hadiza Moussa is gone, tragically killed in a car accident in Niger in 2013. She was not able to pursue her promising work, to continue advising students, all of whom respected her deeply, or to take over the direction of LASDEL in the future. She was my student, then my colleague; and I have still not grown accustomed to her absence from the office next door or from our team discussions. She left a great void, which we all still feel today.

The English translation of this book is therefore unfortunately a posthumous publication, but it is also a last tribute that our team pays her thanks to Alice Kang and Barbara Cooper.

BIBLIOGRAPHY

Cooper, Barbara. 2013. The demographic crisis in the Sahel: what's in a name? *Politique Africaine* 130 (2): 67–88.

Diarra, Aïssa. 2017. Les interruptions volontaires de grossesse au Niger. *Études et travaux du LASDEL* 128: 1–88.

Moussa, Hadiza. 2003a. Niamey: le complexe sanitaire de Boukoki. In *Une médecine inhospitalière. Les difficiles relations entre soignants et soignés dans cinq capitales d'Afrique de l'Ouest*, eds. Yannick Jaffré and Jean-Pierre Olivier de Sardan, 361–385. Paris: Karthala.

Moussa, Hadiza. 2003b. Les pouvoirs locaux à Ngourti. *Études et travaux du LASDEL* 12: 1–47.

Moussa, Hadiza. 2005. Les pouvoirs locaux et le rôle des femmes à Guéladio. *Études et travaux du LASDEL* 36: 1–55.

Moussa, Hadiza. 2007. Les pouvoirs locaux et le rôle des femmes à Guéladio (2). *Études et travaux du LASDEL* 48: 1–38.

Moussa, Hadiza. 2011. Les pouvoirs locaux et le rôle des femmes à Guéladio (4). *Études et travaux du LASDEL* 87: 1–27.

Moussa, Hadiza, and Abdoua Elhadji Dagobi. 2015. Résultats des enquêtes qualitatives sur la santé sexuelle et reproductive des adolescents et des jeunes dans les districts sanitaires d'Aguié et Say. *Études et travaux du LASDEL* 113: 1–95.

Olivier de Sardan, Jean-Pierre. 2015. Practical norms: informal regulations within public bureaucracies (in Africa and beyond). In *Real governance and practical norms in sub-Saharan Africa. The game of the rules*, eds. Tom De Herdt and Jean-Pierre Olivier de Sardan, 19–62. London: Routledge.

Olivier de Sardan, Jean-Pierre. 2017. Rivalries of proximity beyond the household in Niger: political elites and the *baab-izey* pattern. *Africa* 87 (1): 120–136.

Ouédraogo, Ramatou. 2015. L'avortement, ses pratiques et ses soins. Une anthropologie des jeunes au prisme des normes sociales et des politiques publiques de santé au Burkina Faso. PhD diss., Université de Bordeaux.

Ouédraogo, Ramatou, and Agnès Guillaume. 2017. Un désir d'enfant non abouti? Grossesse et avortement chez les jeunes femmes à Ouagadougou (Burkina Faso). *Anthropologie et Sociétés* 41 (2): 39–57.

Peltier, Elian. 2022. A year after widening abortion access, Benin sees fewer botched ones. *The New York Times*, Nov. 13, Section A p. 6.

Sambieni, Emmanuel N'koué, and Elisabeth Paul. 2015. *Analyse comparée des déterminants socioculturels et communautaires des grossesses non désirées et des avortements (Palestine, Pérou, Burkina Faso, République démocratique du Congo).* Paris: LASDEL-Médecins du Monde.

ACKNOWLEDGMENTS

I owe an immense debt to the following: my advisor, Jean-Pierre Olivier de Sardan, who spared no effort during all these years to introduce me to and mentor me in the conduct of rigorous and ethical research; my husband, Moussa Zangaou, who enthusiastically encouraged me to undertake and complete my postgraduate education and supported me in difficult times; Mahamane Tidjani Alou, Doris Bonnet, Yannick Jaffré, Maud Saint-Lary, Abdoua Elhadji Dagobi, and Antoinette Tidjani Alou, who greatly helped me advance my thinking. I wish to express my deep gratitude to each of you.

I thank the Service for Cooperation and Cultural Action of the French Embassy in Niger, LASDEL, and the IRD who helped fund my doctoral studies. I would like to warmly thank the Abdou Moumouni University of Niamey, which provided me the financial support necessary for the publication of this book. I am very grateful to all my friends and colleagues at LASDEL (Niamey and Parakou) for their constant support.

The unending support of my family and friends was critical to the completion of this work. I would particularly like to thank my mother Hadjia Fati Malam Abba, my late father Elhadji Mahaman Fizzan Kedellah, Adama Abdou Zagui, Frédérique Vallaud, and Mohamed Ag Erless.

ACRONYMS

AIDS	Acquired immunodeficiency syndrome
ART	Assisted reproductive technology
CFA	Monetrary unit of the African Financial Community of West African States
CNSR	National Center for Reproductive Health (Centre National de la Santé de la Reproduction)
CPR	Contraceptive prevalence rate
CSI	Full-service health center known as an "integrated health center" (Centre de Santé Intégré)
DSR	Department of Reproductive Health (Direction de la Santé de la Reproduction)
EHESS	École des Hautes Études en Sciences Sociales
GAIPDS	Society of Islamic Associations for Family Planning and Social Development (Groupement des Associations Islamiques en matière de Planification Familiale et Développement Sociale)
GDP	Gross Domestic Product
H	A quotation translated from the Hausa language
HIV	Human immunodeficiency virus
IUD	Intrauterine contraceptive device
LASDEL	Laboratory for Study and Research of Social Dynamics and Local Development (Laboratoire d'Études et de Recherches sur les Dynamiques sociales et le Développement Local)
MIG	Issaka Gazoby Maternity Hospital (Maternité Issaka Gazoby)
NGO	Non-governmental organization
PMI	Maternal and Infant Health Services clinic (Protection Maternelle et Infantile)

SR/PF	Reproductive Health and the Advancement of Women in Islam (Santé de la Reproduction et Promotion de la Femme en Islam)
STD	Sexually transmitted disease
STI	Sexually transmitted infection
UNFPA	United Nations Population Fund (FNUAP)
WHO	World Health Organization
Z	A quotation translated from the Zarma language

Introduction: Infertile Sexuality

This book examines what I call "infertile sexuality"—that is to say, sexual practices and conditions that do not result in procreation. The dominant sexual moral code in much of Africa, particularly evident in Niger, stipulates that married life must lead to the creation of an abundant lineage. Generally, among urban residents and settled agro-pastoralists, infertility, contraception, abortion, and infanticide are all deemed deviant and contrary to mainstream norms and practices. Infertile sexuality in Niger subjects women to social stigma that can range from mild disapproval to severe disapprobation. It is from this socially stigmatized point of entry that I propose to analyze fertility. I address *infertility* and *contraception* to understand how female fertility is managed in the familial, informal, and biomedical spheres. Shedding light on the social practices that control women's bodies and the dynamics these institutions set in motion is crucial to understanding "the governing of the body" (Fassin and Memmi 2004).

Questions related to sexual and reproductive health, and more particularly involving fertility management, are at the heart of demographic, epidemiological, psychological, and public health studies (Caldwell 1982; Caldwell and Caldwell 1987; Pilon and Guillaume 2000; Locoh 1984, 1991). Nevertheless, the regulation of fertility has received very little examination in French-language sociological or anthropological studies in Africa and even less so in the case of Niger. Anthropologist Nicole Echard has shown that in rural Niger gender hierarchies in the 1980s were explicitly founded on women's sexuality. Women learn early to manage their sexuality, seen as the sole capital available to them (Echard 1985: 43). Research on sexual and reproductive health in contemporary Africa tends to focus on three main

Yearning and Refusal. Hadiza Moussa, Edited by Alice J. Kang and Barbara M. Cooper, Oxford University Press.
© Oxford University Press 2023. DOI: 10.1093/oso/9780197662113.003.0001

concerns: childbirth, the AIDS pandemic, and contraception. While there are some doctoral theses written by medical students, academic studies conducted by students at health professional schools, and demographic and epidemiological analyses, no anthropological monograph-length study focusing on fertility has been carried out in Niger. It is this important gap that I seek to redress. I investigate the closely intertwined topics of reproductive health and sexual health through the lens of thwarted fertility.

In Africa and in Niger, the biomedical approach to reproductive health has largely taken over state and parastatal institutions. Outside these formal settings, however, the social management of fertility draws a multitude of less formal social actors together, including the family unit and the extended household, which I refer to as "informal networks." Muslim scholars, therapeutic specialists known as marabouts, traditional healers, and "traveling pharmacists" make up what I refer to as "the popular therapeutic sphere." I use the term "popular" to avoid the reductiveness of the term "traditional," which suggests residual practices from the past.[1] In an urban setting, popular sites of decision-making and therapy management draw upon an eclectic array of materials, ideas, and potencies that are at once contemporary and unofficial.

Fertility is the subject of concerns that go well beyond the interests of the couple alone (Moussa Abdallah 2002). The issue of fertility calls for the consideration of many closely related mechanisms that can affect procreation (sexuality, pregnancy, birth, and breastfeeding), various methods of contraception, and different interventions sought out to prevent and to fight against infertility. Social relationships ordered through gender and generation govern fertility dynamics in ways that privilege the domination of men over women and older individuals over younger ones (Meillassoux 1975).

I begin with the general proposition that, in the city of Niamey, the management of women's fertility occurs in many interconnected social spaces: the socio-familial sphere, the popular therapeutic sphere, and the biomedical sphere. In triggering so many levels of decision-making, the regulation of fertility generates overlapping tensions. In the family circle, reproductive decision-making reinforces the established order by constructing and organizing gendered social relationships. In the medical context, the social relationships between healthcare providers and patients are largely defined by social class. The asymmetrical relationship between them gives

---

1. Editor's note: In French the word *populaire* tends to signal a relatively poor or working-class context, with mass rather than elite allegiance.

rise to friction and hampers the care that women receive. Outside of health centers, the husband, mother, mother-in-law, the extended family, and friends—in short, all those with connections to the married couple— have an intense interest in the proper production of children and in the descendants that the couple has an unconditional obligation to provide. The family parcels out different types of control over fertility to various players in society: traditional healers, marabouts, and biomedical professionals. The regulation of fertility is exercised through the bodies of women.

From this initial point of departure, a number of central observations emerge. First, female fertility is socially managed and supervised only once a woman succeeds in meeting the social prerequisite of maternity. A woman who is pregnant, giving birth, or raising children is almost always supported in these efforts, which confer upon her social recognition of her femininity. Her social existence is defined through and for these tasks. Conversely, infertile women are abandoned to manage their own thwarted fertility more or less independently. A child—"wealth"—generates social symbiosis that is unavailable to the woman who experiences the misfortune of infertility. In her quest for fertility treatment, a woman explores alone the complexities of medical expertise (e.g., consultations and gynecological examinations), as well as the labyrinths and mysteries of common and specialized knowledge in the popular sphere. Infertility is a personal tragedy for women, insofar as they undergo social disgrace and feelings of incompleteness.

Second, the legitimization, choice, and practice of spacing out births give rise to conflict and negotiation within the family circle. Access to biomedical contraception in Niger still requires a challenging "conjugal transaction" for women. Third, women deploy a multitude of stratagems to manage their fertility within the pre-established social landscape. They may use methods that are socially reproved to space out their pregnancies or to render themselves (generally temporarily) infertile.

ANALYZING HUMAN REPRODUCTION IN BOTH ITS BIOLOGICAL AND SOCIAL DIMENSIONS

Because the body is at once biological and social, it offers an interesting point of departure for studying fertility in the social sciences (Bonnet 1988). Carole Browner and Carolyn Sargent note the following:

> Human reproduction is never entirely a biological affair; all societies shape their members' reproductive behavior. This cultural patterning of reproduction

includes the beliefs and practices surrounding menstruation; proscriptions on the circumstances under which pregnancy may occur and who may legitimately reproduce; the prenatal and post-partum practices that mothers-to-be and their significant others observe; the management of labor, the circumstances under which interventions occur, and the form such interventions may take. (1996: 219)

The social dimension of managing women's fertility involves many actors and mechanisms of control.

The study of fertility management invites at least two distinct but interdependent lines of research. The first focuses upon the social production of the desire for children by encouraging procreation as a universal and cosmic necessity and by adopting techniques to fight against infertility. In this approach, the study of fertility addresses maternity, the dysfunctions of the reproductive system relative to infertility, sexual problems that individuals experience, contraceptive practices, and different treatment options. But it must be ever alert to the social ideology surrounding the practices and situations that constitute the diverse forms of expression of reproductive life.

The second line of approach addresses the social control of sexuality as integral to understanding fertility and the mechanisms of human reproduction. The close connection between fertility and sexuality, the former dependent upon the latter (except in the context of certain assisted reproductive technologies [ARTs]), invites reflections on the satisfaction of the objectives of reproduction as an extended process that is always sexual indirectly or directly. As Paola Tabet (1998) insists, the study of fertility calls for attention to the stages of the entire reproductive cycle: sexual socialization; the period of pregnancy, surrounded by an onslaught of interdictions, prescriptions, and norms; potential miscarriage or abortion; childbirth, with its consequent rites; breastfeeding; and, finally, the weaning of the child.

Each stage along a woman's reproductive trajectory constitutes a context for decision-making and for conflict management. Because women's reproductive capacity represents a form of power—the power to ensure social perpetuation—it is a domain that social actors at multiple scales attempt to control in various ways. The control of women's reproductive power often serves the interests of men. In her study of women and patriarchy in the Maghreb, anthropologist Camille Lacoste-Dujardin ([1985] 1996) shows that men often succeed in subtle ways in transferring this task of control and subjugation to other women. Women, therefore, play an essential mediating role in these mechanisms of sexual control. Thus, by way of a "proxy" system, control over the process of human reproduction is exercised by other women—the mother-in-law, aunts, cousins, sisters. These women may be a part of the wife's family or of the husband's. The husband consequently exercises his authority over his wife by way of female intermediaries. The ideology of domination can certainly be shared between men and women.

In this study, the subject of sexuality will be approached as coterminous with that of fertility. Michel Foucault presents sexuality as an ensemble of "practices, representations, and knowledge" that may be analyzed as a "political apparatus" "acting on the body" (1986). By this way of thinking, fertility management, via sexuality, entails political control, both in the form of an "obligation to comply" on the part of women's bodies and through mental subjugation. Similarly, Tabet argues that the management of human reproduction is underpinned by "the search for hegemony in politico-social matters," which calls for the management of women's bodies: "control over reproduction passes necessarily through the preliminary control over women's sexuality" (1998: 151).

If in Niger we celebrate "normal" forms of expression of reproductive life through procreation, what happens in cases of infertility? How are infertile women, or those who—for a certain period—decline to take on motherhood, perceived in Niger and, more specifically, in Niamey? Does the burden of non-birth fall entirely on the woman in a couple? Does a woman's possible treatment entail the intervention of the husband and other members of the extended family?

THE SOCIAL CONTROL OF FERTILITY: INFERTILITY AND CONTRACEPTION

Because of the breadth and complexity of the question of fertility management, I investigate certain aspects of fertility more than others. In focusing upon thwarted fertility, I attend less to pregnancy, birth, and breastfeeding than to infertility management and contraceptive practices. I offer the most detailed ethnography possible of the emic conceptions and practices surrounding the social control of female fertility in the urban context of Niamey, Niger. The individuals involved belong to different sociocultural milieus structured along urban lines; their agency is framed by urban possibilities and constraints often imbued with their own interpretations of biomedical understandings of conception and reproduction.

My work takes two principal lines of inquiry through focused empirical research. The first line of inquiry, involuntary infertility, addresses the social expectations, representations, and practices of procreation in the family circle, particularly with regard to the married couple. In the first half of the book, I consider the socially institutionalized relationships between sexual and reproductive life. Social perceptions regarding procreation govern attitudes toward any malfunction of the female reproductive system. In this regard, an empirical study of people's common knowledge about infertility, their preventative practices, and the strategies they use and share to counter the "reproductive anxiety" that infertility provokes is necessary. Only through an anthropological study of affect in the context of the lived experience and quotidian sensations of infertile individuals is it truly possible to understand the dual embodied concepts of successful birth and reproductive failure.

The second axis concerns contraception. In *A History of Contraception: From Antiquity to the Present Day*, Angus McLaren emphasizes that the desire for reproductive control is universal (1990). This impulse to regulate fertility nevertheless varies according to sociocultural contexts. To understand contraceptive practices, one must situate them in their social environments. The second half of this book examines the actual practice of contraception in Niamey in all its forms. Above all, it endeavors to show that contraceptive fertility management sits at the crossroads of quite different norms: "official" familial objections to the idea of spacing births, on the one hand, and medical and individual advice more inclined to promote "rational" fertility regulation, on the other hand. I describe and analyze the uses of the various contraceptive treatments employed in the city of Niamey and its surroundings, ranging from "grandmother" recipes to popular therapies to biomedical interventions. Contraceptive practice in Niger, whatever the form, is a matter of tricky navigation on the part of users. Women negotiate access to contraception to moderate tensions within or outside the home, with relatives, or in health centers. I explore some of the microstrategies women employ to sidestep social constraints. I also address the most "extreme" case of contraception (as my respondents characterized it): that of married women who turn to abortion. Contraceptive abortions reveal the deep ambiguities of conjugal, familial, and social relationships.

What are the linkages between the conjugal, popular, and medical regulation of reproduction in these two contexts—that of managing infertility and seeking contraception? Urban life in Niger demands a multitude of incompatible actions, practices, and status behaviors of women. Women must balance all these in managing their sexual and reproductive lives.

NORMATIVE MARRIAGE AND SEXUALITY: THE CONJUGAL DEBT

Before turning to the exploration of infertility and contraception, it will be useful for me to provide an overview of the normative framework against which infertile sexuality is measured. In Niger, marriage is the only legitimate context for sexuality. As one marabout put it, "God codified sexuality for married people. For those who aren't married, this is an issue that doesn't concern them. It's because of marriage that God gave men sexuality—without marriage, no sexuality" (Malam I, 51 years old, Bagdad district).[2] It must also be said that how one expresses one's sexuality is rarely discussed, even within this legitimate context. Conjugal sexuality, despite its omnipresence in women's lives, is absent from everyday language. It is as if a strong and tacit rule states, "Have sex, but don't talk about it." The incommunicability of sexuality is, as we can see, a social requirement that applies much more strictly to women.

In Niger, there is both great flexibility and unequivocal ambiguity in social standards according to sex. It goes without saying that the material consequences of pre-marital sex for women (defloration and pregnancy) are easy to observe. As hard and intangible, as categorical and rigid as these norms are for women, they offer great flexibility to men. For girls, the obligation of virginity in a bride is emphasized as a non-negotiable and repressive requirement. A new bride's virginity remains a matter of honor for all parties involved in the marriage. Yet this ethos is defended and appropriated differently by each family because it is for the girl's family and for her mother in particular that virginity represents an opportunity for personal and familial moral enhancement; it is proof of the mother's dignity. A girl who is not a virgin is necessarily debauched. She is perceived as such "because her mother did not know how to educate her well." During the weeks devoted to wedding ceremonies, the moment most dreaded by young brides is undoubtedly the day after the wedding night. The family network, friends, and curious bystanders converge at the bride's family home and at the young groom's home to find out if the bride "stained" the clean white linen that was placed on the wedding mattress.

More than the rupture of the hymen, parents fear pre-marital pregnancy which demands far more complicated management than that of virginity as it manifests the prohibited sexual practice more explicitly. Despite the importance of virginity and the avoidance of pre-marital pregnancy, the strong social censorship of speaking about sex means that parents

---

2. *Malam* and *alpha* are generic terms used to describe marabouts, in Hausa and Zarma, respectively.

spend little energy on sex education. For some parents, broaching sexuality with their children is a formidable ordeal, even when their children are old enough to marry. The absence of sexual socialization is so strong that many mothers find it inappropriate to talk to their daughters about menstruation. When parents approach their children's puberty, they avoid going into anatomical and physiological details and simply describe the period as "dangerous." Accordingly, menstrual blood often comes as a surprise. Girls are caught off guard, although some learn from older siblings, friends, or classmates.

Islam identifies marital sex (*nikâh* in Arabic) as a form of sacrament, of transcendence by way of carnal relations (Bouhdiba 2001: 113). Within this framework, sexuality takes the form of a duty commonly referred to as "conjugal duty" or "conjugal debt."[3] The obligation to perform the sexual act is equal for each spouse: the wife must not "close her loincloth" or "tie the bed," and the husband must respect this religious injunction. In reality, however, there is a strong feminization of the marital debt. It is in fact the woman who is often reminded that refusing to have marital sex is a serious sin. A woman who does not fulfill her conjugal duty will be cursed, perhaps saved from the gates of hell only if her husband forgives her, according to my interviews with marabouts. The feminization of the conjugal debt may have developed prior to Christianity and Islam. In the context of this study, one can hypothesize that it worsened with the advent of Islam.

Not once in my investigation did the women I met mention their own pleasure; rather, they mentioned only that of men. Women deploy considerable resources to satisfy their husbands, while the reverse is not widely true. Simply put, women put a lot of energy into making themselves desirable to their husbands. In general, women think it necessary to maximize their sexual performance at all costs to feel closer, more loved by their partner. Affective failure can lead to the arrival of a co-wife or prompt a divorce. In monogamous households, women do everything in their power to prevent their husbands from wandering and to guard against the intrusion of co-wives. Similarly, in polygamous households, co-wives engage in "conjugal guerrilla" tactics to rid themselves of competition.

This feminized conjugal debt goes well beyond sexual obligations and the competition of co-wives. In addition to submitting to her husband, the bride must be unconditionally at the service of his relatives and friends. The new bride wife must "take care of them" so as not to run the risk of

3. Derived from the Latin *debitum conjugale*.

upsetting the marital balance. This powerful social context sets the stage for the experience of infertile sexuality explored in the chapters to follow.

GLOBAL REPRODUCTIVE HEALTH IN NIGER

The concept of "reproductive health" has been on the rise since the end of the 1980s (Bonnet and Guillaume 1999). With its promise of promoting development, reproductive health and its corollaries—"reproductive rights," "responsible parenting," "safe motherhood," and "safe sex"—occupy the public and semi-public policy spheres around the world. This is particularly palpable in third world countries like Niger. National institutions—strongly urged on by development agencies such as the United Nations Population Fund (UNFPA), United Nations Children's Fund, as well as international non-governmental organizations (NGOs)—seek to implement international reproductive health resolutions.

International organizations increasingly guide decision-making discourses regarding the promotion of reproductive health via public and semi-public institutions (NGOs, development projects, and civil society associations). Niger has a national reproductive health policy in conformity with the resolutions of the 1994 Cairo Conference. The reproductive health policy comprises nine priority objectives: the advancement of health for all, control over fertility, risk-free maternity, family planning, combatting sexually transmitted infections/HIV/AIDS, care for children under the age of five, care for adolescents, combatting genital cancers and reproductive afflictions, and improvement of the physical, socioeconomic, and cultural environment. Niger has instituted the Department of Reproductive Health (Direction de la Santé de la Reproduction [DSR]) to implement the policy. The DSR oversees at the national level the different elements of the reproductive health program, which in line with the UN Population Fund recommendations seeks "to promote women's and children's health, as well as that of men" (FNUAP, 2000). The creation of the National Center for Reproductive Health (Centre National de la Santé de la Reproduction [CNSR]) as well as the modernization and increase in patient capacity at the Central Maternity Hospital in Niamey have stemmed from the same objective.

The mainstream approach to reproductive health considers fertility to be the business of women alone. Although academic circles are today more or less aware of this bias, in the daily life of healthcare structures and NGOs, programs are still attached to this principle that excludes the man, neglecting the socially constructed character of the management of women's fertility and of all the practices that surround it. What is problematic is both the exclusion of men from reproductive health and the single-minded focus on birth control.

DEMOGRAPHICS OF NIGER

According to the 2001 census results, the population of Niger is 11,060,291 (Bureau Central du Recensement 2005). The distribution of people across the country's eight regions is Agadez (2.9%), Diffa (3.1%), Dosso (13.6%), Maradi (20.2%), Niamey (6.4%), Tahoua (17.9%), Tillabery (17.1%), and Zinder (18.8%). While overall Niger's population density is 8.7 inhabitants per square kilometer, some regions such as Dosso (in the west) and Maradi (in the center-east) register 44.5 and 53.5 inhabitants per square kilometer. By contrast, in Agadez (to the north) and Diffa (in the east), these figures are 0.5 and 2.2, respectively (Figure I.1).

Niger's total fertility rate is the highest not only in sub-Saharan Africa but also in the world (Attama et al. 1998; UNFPA 2000). Niger's population has an annual increase of 3.3%. Fertility rates in Niger remain high despite

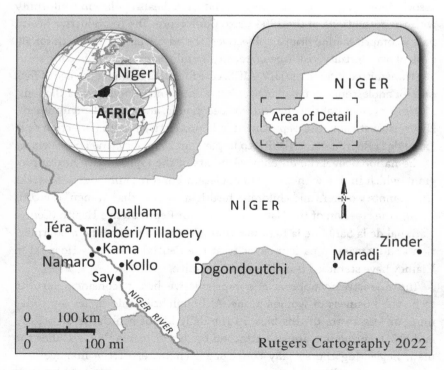

Figure I.1 Map of Niger

the presence of family planning services in the country for more than two decades. A married Nigerien woman who has reached the end of her reproductive years (45–49 years) has given birth to an average of 7.1 children (Institute National de la Statistique 2006).[4] Fertility in Niger begins early and is long and intense. Marriages in rural areas occur at a relatively young age—often younger than 15 for girls, which leads to early motherhood. The contraceptive prevalence rate remains low, at approximately 11.2% (5% for biomedical methods and 6.2% for traditional methods). Pregnancies generally only end when menopause is reached. The multiple consequences of early childbearing in Niger include miscarriage, premature birth, perineal tearing, fistula and infections that can cause infertility, low birth weight, and cervical cancer (CERPOD 1996).

Niger's strong pro-natal tendency is in large part driven by the country's high infant mortality rate. Many infants die before the age of one year. The infant mortality rate is estimated to be 123 deaths per 1,000 children less than one year old.[5] This rate is higher in rural areas where women, who often suffer the loss of their own children or are worried by this phenomenon, maximize the number of their pregnancies in anticipation of losing a child (Moussa 2003).

Alongside Niger's high infant mortality rate are elevated levels of maternal mortality. Approximately 652 women die for reasons related to childbirth or pregnancy per 100,000 live births according to UNFPA (2000).[6] The high mortality results, on the one hand, from a high prevalence of infectious and endemo-epidemic diseases (particularly measles and malaria) and, on the other hand, from a low vaccination coverage rate for women of childbearing age. Inadequate prenatal care affects both infants and their mothers. Postpartum problems for women include damage to the uterus, infections, obstetric hemorrhages, and nutritional anemia. Attending to a birth in Niger, whether in a medical center or not, is a particularly difficult task. The persistence of food insecurity also affects the nutritional status of all vulnerable groups including young children, breastfeeding women, and pregnant women. The progression of sexually transmitted diseases from 1980 to 2000 rapidly increased the

4. Editor's note: According to UNFPA (2022), Niger's population size in 2021 is estimated at 25,100,000, with a growth rate of 3.3% and a fertility rate of 6.6 children per woman.

5. Editor's note: This estimate fell to 46.7 per 1,000 live births in 2019 but remains relatively high compared with other countries in the region (United Nations Interagency Group for Child Mortality Estimation 2021).

6. Editor's note: Approximately 509 maternal deaths per 100,000 live births in 2017 (Global Health Observatory 2019).

number of new HIV/AIDS cases per annum from eight in 1989 to a peak of approximately 3,600 in 1998 (UNFPA 2000). AIDS continues to disrupt the healthcare landscape; but the situation is far more stable today, and mother–infant transmission is preventable.[7] All of these combined affects the average life expectancy, which was estimated in 2000 to be less than 50 years (48.4 years).

Approximately half (48%) of the population is younger than 15 years. Beyond the family circle, the vulnerable situation of mothers and children has garnered the attention of public and scientific leaders. This concern manifests itself in population development programs. Because of its importance both in the continuation of the community and to population-related policy, worries about population growth have prompted intervention by numerous public and semi-public institutions.

My research site, Niamey, is the capital of Niger. The population of Niamey in 2001 was approximately 1,026,848 inhabitants (Bureau Central du Recensement 2004). Like other capital cities, Niamey is cosmopolitan. Its population includes all of Niger's ethnic groups, as well as numerous sociolinguistic groups from the West African region (e.g., Benin, Burkina Faso, Côte d'Ivoire, Mali, Nigeria, Senegal). This highly diverse urban population might lead one to expect a wide range of attitudes, representations, practices, and symbols surrounding procreation. While a range of practices exist, the value assigned to childbirth is widely, if not universally, shared. There is a pronounced convergence in points of view and aspirations: legal conjugal unions must result in childbirth.

AN ETHNOGRAPHY OF FERTILITY MANAGEMENT: RESEARCH METHODS

Understanding fertility in Niger requires attention to the social construction of fertility in the familial, popular, and biomedical realms. The anthropology of fertility must examine the convergences and contradictions between these spheres as they affect the regulation of women's reproductive lives. My research has been iterative and multifaceted, juxtaposing interviews with observations, norms with practices, and documents with lived reality.

---

7. Editor's note: According to UNAIDS (2020), Niger's HIV prevalence rate among adults aged 15–49 is a relatively low 0.2.

Study Sites

I sought to understand national policy as it relates to reproductive health and medical training but also to grasp the on-the-ground medical management of fertility and the kinds of social interactions that it entailed. I conducted interviews and observations at three major maternity centers (Central Maternity Hospital, Talladjé Maternity Ward, and Boukoki Maternity Ward); two maternal and infant health services clinic (*protection maternelle et infantile* [PMI]) centers, in Gaweye and Lamordé; and the CNSR (Figure I.2). Discussing fertility and infertility with health workers (midwives, social workers, nurses, gynecologists, and obstetricians) helped shed light on the different types of technical and non-technical interventions (psychological, for instance) that the medical establishment enacts upon women, in particular during the treatment of infertility. The Central Maternity Hospital and the CNSR are the two referral sites for sexual and reproductive health and are therefore equipped with modern technical resources. The Talladjé and Boukoki sites are located in districts farther from downtown Niamey and are heavily frequented. Patients who use them typically have modest incomes.

Niamey's Central Maternity Hospital, renamed Maternité Issaka Gazoby in 1997 after one of its most illustrious gynecologists and obstetricians, is the national referral hospital for the management of complex gynecological and obstetrical cases. The Central Maternity Hospital also serves as a teaching hospital for medical students, midwives, and paramedics. Each year, the center welcomes many student trainees from the major medical training institutions (National School of Public Health [École Nationale de Santé Publique], School of Public Health and Social Work [Ecole de Santé Publique et de l'Action Sociale], Practical Training Institute of Public Health [Institut Pratique de Santé Publique], Institute of Public Health [Institut de Santé Publique], and Advanced Institute of Public Health [Institut Supérieur de Santé Publique]). In 2007, the Central Maternity Hospital had 206 employees, including 27 administrative executives, 13 doctors (eight of whom were gynecologists-obstetricians), 40 midwives, 19 nurses, and five social workers. To increase its technical capacity, the hospital was equipped with a mammography unit in 2003. Additionally, representatives have been sent abroad for training in preparation of offering ART services.

The Talladjé Maternity Ward is part of the integrated health center (*centre de santé intégré*) that bears the same name. The Talladjé district is located on the outskirts of the city and is part of the Niamey II commune. According to the 2001 census, its population was around 35,000. Talladjé is a working-class neighborhood inhabited largely by populations with

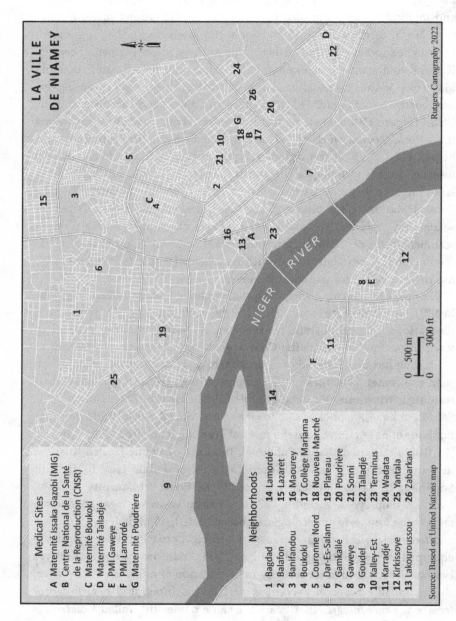

Medical Sites

A Maternité Issaka Gazobi (MIG)
B Centre National de la Santé
  de la Reproduction (CNSR)
C Maternité Boukoki
D Maternité Talladjé
E PMI Gaweye
F PMI Lamordé
G Maternité Poudrière

Neighborhoods

1 Bagdad
2 Balafon
3 Banifandou
4 Boukoki
5 Couronne Nord
6 Dar-Es-Salam
7 Gamkallé
8 Gaweye
9 Goudel
10 Kalley-Est
11 Karradjé
12 Kirkissoye
13 Lakouroussou
14 Lamordé
15 Lazaret
16 Maourey
17 Collège Mariama
18 Nouveau Marché
19 Plateau
20 Poudrière
21 Sonni
22 Talladjé
23 Terminus
24 Wadata
25 Yantala
26 Zabarkan

LA VILLE
DE NIAMEY

NIGER RIVER

0   500 m
0   3000 ft

Rutgers Cartography 2022

Source: Based on United Nations map

Figure I.2 Map of Study Sites

mostly low incomes and a few wealthy families who have settled there in recent years because of the housing crisis in the city center. The complex also includes a free clinic and a PMI center. The maternity ward consists of 12 post-delivery beds. The staff is composed of 11 midwives, one obstetric technician, four laborers, four civil registry personnel, one driver, and 10 room attendants (including one volunteer). The hospital's principal activities are childbirth, prevention of mother-to-child transmission, obstetrics and gynecology consultations, and the establishment of vital records.

I also conducted observations and interviews in "unofficial" spaces. These included, importantly, the family. In the households I was interested not only in the conjugal relationship but also in the rest of the extended family (thought of locally in terms of lineage) and other close domestic relationships. In the popular sphere I interviewed actors versed in the magico-religious tradition (marabouts, traditional healers), as well as street vendors of various products (pharmaceuticals, aphrodisiacs, and other sexual stimulants). The former were interviewed most often at their homes and market stalls. I sought out the latter in the three main locations where they operate: bus stations, areas around markets, and near healthcare facilities.

I began learning the lay of the land for this project in November 2002 to January 2003. This preliminary research phase involved identifying the main actors—the people and institutions concerned with the management of fertility. In this initial round of data collection and assessment, I was able to define the research problem in more detail and develop interview guides. Importantly, during this phase, I became more acutely aware of the methodological challenges in studying infertility (which I address in the next section). It was during this period that my theoretical and methodological foundation developed.

The fieldwork itself unfolded in three waves. The first wave lasted five months, from February to June 2003, during which time I focused on visiting medical centers. I then conducted a second series of interviews and observations between August 2004 and the end of January 2005, focusing on the family and the popular sphere with an emphasis on infertility. During this period, I focused on tracing individual women's therapeutic journeys, from family planning or infertility consultations to either traditional healers (often referred to in French as "fetishists") or marabouts and often street vendors and, of course, in marital or other family structures. In a final field phase from September 2005 to February 2006, I focused on women's contraceptive practices. After February 2006, I often returned to the field to clarify or deepen the pieces of information I had gathered.

My interviews, which were extensive and often recorded, were translated and transcribed in their entirety. This enabled me to collect "discursive data giving access to emic representations of respondents" (Olivier de Sardan 1995: 81). These data were split into several categories ranging from ordinary interviews to biographies or life stories to the formation of case studies. In conducting interviews at multiple sites in Niamey, I sought to reconstruct the trajectories of women as they encountered their families, traditional healers and marabouts, health centers, and public policy in their pursuit of managing their fertility. Some women who had no children, and could be classified as sterile, I followed for three years.

Most often, I first encountered women in a medical setting, during consultations (see Table I.1). Interviews in that initial setting were often not particularly productive, whether with healthcare personnel or patients. For the latter group, a change of scenery was very beneficial in the sense that interviewees felt more at ease in their homes, far from the intimidation (real or perceived) experienced at the maternity ward, PMI center, or CNSR. To supplement on-site observations of interactions in medical environments, I conducted home interviews with certain patients. This proved to be a difficult undertaking in the beginning, in part because I had not yet entirely understood the consequences of family intrusions into the decision-making process concerning contraceptive use or the treatment of

Table I.1 SUMMARY OF INTERVIEWS

Strategic groups	Characteristics of respondents	Interviews
Informal networks	Women attending consultations	27
	Women interviewed at home	23
	Members of the close circle (spouses, relatives, friends, companions)	21
Popular therapeutic sphere	Marabouts	11
	Traditional healers	9
	(Itinerant) Street vendors	7
Institutional structures	Healthcare providers	17
	Ministry, NGO, and other association officials	6
Other groups	Adolescents, *foyandi* participants	5
Total		**126**

infertility. I also observed and interviewed women in the *foyandi* (Z) social groups where women (married and single) meet to share meals and contribute to an informal savings bank called *asusu*.[8]

I make no claim that this sample is representative of all women. These cases constitute individual journeys as much as commonly experienced situations. They illustrate an essential theme set forth throughout this work: that the social construction of femininity in Niger occurs only through motherhood. In local constructions, femininity and motherhood are intertwined in such a way that one takes on its meaning in relation to the other. Setting out multiple different portraits of women with fertility conditions offers the advantage of bringing together a range of experiences across social circles that nevertheless overlap—they are separate, but they are not isolated. Their stories reveal the twists and turns, good or bad, that characterize their sexual and reproductive trajectories, as well as the battles they fought to improve their status as "childless women."

Because I was interested in conjugal relations, I attempted to speak not just with married women but also with their husbands individually and as couples. Seeking out the men's point of view widens our understanding of the management of fertility by highlighting the social relationships surrounding sex. This approach has generally been underexplored by demographers of Niger. Interviewing a husband and wife together was not an easy task. Even when the idea of a couple's interview was accepted, some men left before the interview was over, leaving the wife alone with the researcher.

Since fertility regulation also involves other members of the lineage, my effort to understand fertility in the domestic sphere was widened to include discussions with the extended family (e.g., mothers, mothers-in-law, aunts, sisters, and brothers). Marabouts, traditional healers, and itinerant vendors, because of their place at the forefront of the popular management of fertility, provided information on their practices, their customers, and their positioning in the general therapeutic market. Finally, I interviewed elders, particularly older women who were known to be skilled in matters related to fertility and childbirth, to learn about earlier types of fertility management and how they have changed.

8. This bank provides emergency funds with low interest rates (5%–10%) to members who request them. More generally, *foyandi* corresponds to the day of rest following a marriage or naming. The verb *foy* means "to pass the middle of the day" (Bernard and White-Kaba 1994: 106).

Observations

Many of the interviews were combined with observations (see Table I.2). Seeing real interactions within health structures (PMI centers, maternity wards, and hospitals) led me to take an interest in the trajectories of specific women (both with and without children). Inside the healthcare centers, I attended different kinds of consultation sessions, from gynecological appointments to address infertility to post-natal check-ups, to family planning visits. I focused here because these moments, together with assisted deliveries, are the most decisive in determining methods of fertility regulation imposed upon or offered to women attending health clinics. In addition to being present at some of my interviewees' health consultations, I made observations when I visited their homes. During all these instances, I took detailed descriptive notes that were then coded. I have favored a Goffmanian perspective, in which the rites of interaction are meticulously described and reported.

The observational method has several limitations. My presence in health centers was sometimes considered to be intrusive, particularly in light of a previous team's investigation that healthcare providers deemed too critical. Anthropological investigation seemed to some medical workers to be a kind of malicious inquisition rather than an effort to further scientific understanding. In the home environment, it is not easy to discern all the hidden ways that a woman's family members influence decisions regarding her health (for treating possible infertility and for using contraception). While on-site observations of interactions between caregivers and patients provide a relatively unfiltered kind of evidence, unlike interviews, certain fertility-related and sexual practices, particularly if they are illegal, cannot be reconstructed through observation (Bozon 1995; Elias 1973; Koster 2003).

Table I.2 SUMMARY OF OBSERVATIONS

Context or nature of observation	Number of observations
Appointments and consultations	21
Following a patient through multiple encounters at a health center	4
Births	3
Marriage ceremonies	3
Baptisms	2
Foyandi meetings	2
Household visits	6
Total	**41**

In the very early phases of carrying out this study, I found myself asking and giving considerable thought to who I am as a researcher. This was the first difficulty I encountered in the field: my unease with studying the management of women's fertility and its related topics (e.g., social relations, sex, sexuality, religious socialization, family planning). Certainly, the researcher can learn the local codes of decorum (Olivier de Sardan 1995: 74). Indeed, they are the very codes that govern my own life as a resident of Niamey. But how does one study taboo subjects such as the sexual aspects of fertility? In my field sites, the social code prohibits speaking about sexuality either directly or indirectly. Violating this proscription indicates a bad upbringing, especially for girls and women.

Being an "endo-ethnologist" does not necessarily make doing this research easier. I sometimes wondered whether being Nigerien might not make it harder. Many people in Niamey, particularly women, find it easier to talk about their sexual experiences or are more neutral about sexual matters in general with an outsider, particularly a European or American *annasara* ([Z] a White person), rather than with someone from within their own sociocultural milieu (Olivier de Sardan 1995, 2000; Ouattara 2004). In a small city such as Niamey, a researcher "at home" may discover a kinship connection to an interviewee or find that they are in the same social network. To avoid the issues of interviewing certain respondents that I was overly familiar with, I sometimes sought the help of a research assistant, Fatima Diouldé. She conducted eight interviews with healthcare workers who I knew well or who were schoolmates of mine. I also did not interview my own doctor. This mitigated the possibility of certain biases. I also found that I had to impose a certain self-censorship to dispel the potential for embarrassment for one party or the other in interviews.

My work came up against three main problems that arise because of the taboo nature of the subject of fertility. First, in medical and administrative settings in Niger, fertility is generally conceived of in demographic and epidemiological terms (birth rate, mortality, infertility, or family planning) with quantitative indicators. The various social mechanisms implemented to regulate fertility are often obscured in the rhetoric of many clinic workers and health officials. An obsession with figures often prevailed in the responses to my questions. Caregivers often believe they have a duty to provide numbers on attendance, recovery, and hospitalization rates, instead of observations about practices, ideas, interactions, or decision-making processes.

Second, my own femininity shaped my interactions. On the one hand, my experiences as a woman, a patient, and a wife made it difficult to be objective. At certain stages, the abstract theme "fertility management" seemed impossible to approach with the necessary detachment. Investigating the management of fertility in Niamey placed me face to face with myself, my story, my own journey as a Nigerien woman who has internalized the very standards I sought to question and analyze. On the other hand, being a Nigerien woman, born and raised in Niamey, does give me a deep familiarity with questions of family life.

Social and religious norms, societal representations about sexuality, and one's own personal history are weighty and difficult to disentangle. Aware of this fact, I was at times uncomfortable with some interviewees as it is difficult to address issues related to pregnancy without implicitly referring to the sexual act. The terms that I initially used to refer to fertility were of rather limited scientific and practical use. Given that the term "fertility" covers a range of sub-themes, limiting oneself to speaking just about motherhood renders an analysis very incomplete.

My solution to this methodological challenge was to break the concept of fertility into its various components (sexual relations, desire, pleasure, male and female genitalia, motherhood, infertility, family planning, abortion). I was sometimes accused implicitly and explicitly of abusing the codes of social propriety that conceal these issues that provoke such embarrassment and modesty. In view of the subject's delicate nature and of the prevailing social norms in a strongly Islamized society, there was a danger to both researcher and informant of being stigmatized for deviating from conventions. One 50-year-old woman accused me of not respecting the socio-religious prescriptions and proscriptions that impose modesty and restraint on women. The clear message I was given was that fertility and its mechanisms are "inappropriate" subjects. Although I am fluent in Hausa and Zarma, I nevertheless did experience misunderstandings that caused me to "lose face" in the Goffmanian sense. I quickly learned that in any spoken interaction adhering to implicit rules and conventions is crucial for each of the actors.

SEMIOLOGY AS AN ELEMENT OF THE ETHNOGRAPHIC METHOD

Certain semiological tools did help to break this deadlock. Circumlocution proved to be useful in naming practices banned from common speech or in referring to shameful body parts. The terms presented constitute the vocabulary of common manners, which quite naturally excludes terms and expressions considered coarse or vulgar. Thus, for example, female genitalia become in Hausa *katsa ta* ("one's lower part") or *abunta* ("one's thing") and in Zarma *wayborataray* (literally, "one's femininity"). The female sexual organ is also indicated in Zarma by the phrase *irkoy dia cito*, or "the Prophet's buttonhole" (Diarra 1971). Sexual intercourse becomes *cere diyan* ("encounter") or *marguyan* ("union") in Zarma, and it becomes *tarawa* ("union") or *yin sunna* ("to perform sunna") in Hausa. *Yin sunna* refers to following practices in the tradition of the Prophet Mohammed (the *sunna*), in which it is said that the sexual act is sacred (Bouhdiba 2001). To engage in conjugal intercourse is therefore an act of salvation conforming to a divine prescription.

In local languages, expressions that refer to the act of defloration, generally considered in an extra- and more precisely pre-conjugal context, emphasize the idea of alteration. It is said of a girl who has lost her virginity *a sara* or *a hasara* (Z) and *ta baace* or *ta lalace* (H), all of which mean "she is spoiled." It is possible to convey the responsibility of a man or boy as agent (*a na sara/a na hasara* [Z] or *ya lalatata* [H], "he spoiled her"); however—significantly—the perpetrator is rarely referred to in this way. The main focus is on the deviant character of the girl "who allowed herself to be taken," "who showed her poor upbringing," or "who is a *gabdi*" (seductress, tease, woman of loose morals [Z]).

Throughout this book I focus systematically upon the semiology of sexuality and reproduction not only because such conventions facilitated communication but also because my reflections on semiotics drew out the underlying dynamics and perceptions that shape women's sense of their own standing and the kinds of choices available to them.

OUTLINE OF THE BOOK

I have structured this work into three parts.[9] Part I (Chapters 1–4) examines the social construction of female infertility and how it affects women's lives. In Chapter 1, I set out the dominant norms and values of sexuality and fertility in Niger before discussing the infertile body and the social representations that surround it. Then, in Chapter 2, I discuss the prevention of infertility and locally sought-out treatments to combat it. I also lay out socially appropriate methods for coping with infertility, which include polygamy and child fostering.

9. Editor's note: We have revised this section to reflect the presentation of chapters in the English edition of the book.

Next, in Chapter 3, I present the trajectories of six women who have not known the "ultimate blessing" of producing children, following them into their family settings, popular health networks, and the medical sphere. These women have distinctly contrasting destinies but are socially cast as "childless women." In the spirit of Yannick Jaffré's ethnographic work, Chapter 4 offers an anthropological study of emotion that emerges out of the case studies in Chapter 3. Throughout Part I, I discuss how studying infertility serves as a foundation to understand the social dynamics governing female fertility.

Part II (Chapter 5) of the book provides a critical evaluation of women's experiences at clinics and hospitals in Niamey. I identify challenges and tensions that arise for women desiring treatment for infertility and for women seeking to use biomedical contraception.

The last part of the book, Part III (Chapters 6–8), analyzes contraception in all its aspects, particularly through my conversations with women about their contraceptive knowledge, use, and practices, as well as the paths that lead them to use it (Chapters 6 and 7). Contraceptive practices, which have a bearing on numerous interlocking social issues, create conflict but also give rise to negotiations between a multitude of social actors: between patients and medical personnel (as discussed in Chapter 5), between patients and social actors in the informal care networks (Chapter 6), and between married couples, sexes, and individuals and their community (Chapter 7). Induced abortion as a form of contraception is the subject of Chapter 8.

PART I

The Problem of Infertility

CHAPTER 1

The Infertile Body

In my interviews people regularly repeated the phrase, "There is no worldly wealth as important as having a wealth of children." Jean Bodin's famous dictum "the only real wealth is people" continues to capture the reality shared by a large part of humanity. This sentiment is deeply ingrained and respected in many African societies, including those in Niger. When unable to produce children, the individual often experiences desolation and sadness (Retel-Laurentin 1974). Some women have not become pregnant for lack of ovulation, for lack of a "good partner," due to certain previously contracted illnesses, or for reasons that remain mysterious.

This chapter discusses popular understandings of the infertile body and the social representations that surround it. In Niamey, the primary urban center of Niger, "traditional" and "modern" conceptions of fertility and infertility intersect. But more influential than the rationalizing views of the medical and scientific world are superstitions and symbolic representations circulating as popular beliefs that require attention. I begin by addressing the disproportionate burden of guilt placed upon women in the attribution of blame for a couple's infertility. I will then address the symbolism of infertility, the semiology commonly attached to it, and the "popular hermeneutics" of sterility.

A WOMAN'S STERILITY: THE A PRIORI IMPUTATION OF GUILT

LB and I stayed married for six years. After being married for four and a half years, we hadn't been able to have children and we ended up separating. I'd started to consult marabouts and healers as early as the eighth month [of marriage].

Yearning and Refusal. Hadiza Moussa, Edited by Alice J. Kang and Barbara M. Cooper, Oxford University Press.
© Oxford University Press 2023. DOI: 10.1093/oso/9780197662113.003.0002

I went to the CNSR [National Center for Reproductive Health] starting in the fourteenth month. There, they prescribed products to take for one trimester. At the end of the treatment, I went back to see them. The doctor examined my tubes—there was nothing wrong with them. After that he prescribed another trimester-long treatment that didn't do anything. It was after this second treatment that he asked me to come back with my husband, who was preparing to get married [to a second wife]. We were in our twenty-third month of marriage. He refused to respond to the doctor's request because his mother had told him that I wouldn't be able to have a child, that I'd had two years to prove it. She's sure I'm sterile. Her confidence is reinforced by the fact that her son doesn't have *impuissance* [erectile dysfunction]. So she forced my husband to take another wife. My co-wife left the house after 11 months. Despite this new development, my husband said he wasn't responsible. He remarried again, but even after our divorce he still hadn't had any children. (Madame BB, 29 years old, remarried, mother of one child, Couronne Nord district)

Many women have recounted to me their husband's opposition to seeking diagnosis or treatment for themselves. The great difficulty of encouraging men to take responsibility when a couple experiences infertility (when the man does not suffer from erectile dysfunction) is an issue that regularly came out in my interviews. Even before any medical diagnosis or magico-religious divination, it is the woman who is first suspected of being the cause of a couple's infertility. The possibility of a man being infertile, although recognized, is only considered as a last resort. Social pressures weigh quite unevenly on the two spouses. Men benefit from the disproportionate attention placed on maternity as opposed to paternity.

The concealment of male sterility is so common in my study sample that in every case the first palliative steps were taken by the woman. The case of Madame HZ1, a 39-year-old woman is an example. Madame HZ1's husband took 11 years to be convinced of and to recognize his sterility. She divorced him immediately after this late recognition, and it took her two years to remarry. But nature seemed to tell her it was too late. The time threshold set by age was no longer in her favor. Madame HZ1, who had initially showed no clinical signs of infertility, subsequently struggled to produce viable eggs due to her age.

The joint management of infertility by the couple is thus compromised from the start. The purported absence of male infertility is closely linked to the difficulty of establishing the biological paternity of the child. There is no masculine parallel to the visible biological experience of maternity, upon which the maturation of a woman's status depends. While maternity—that is, biological maternity—does not lend itself to any

falsification or distortion, paternity is always ambiguous and often subject to debate.

> When a child is born, there's no doubt who the mother is, but that's not always
> the case with the father. It's quite simple: we see the mother giving birth to
> the child, the father, no. (Madame HF, 59 years old, retired midwife, Talladjé
> district)

This focus on women is even more pronounced in health centers, where
examinations or surgical procedures are sometimes prescribed to women
unnecessarily. The ability to have an erection, an obvious sign of virility,
protects men from preliminary investigations and questions about the
couple's infertility. Even if the man is not immediately and absolutely
excluded from the treatment plan, the doctor never insists from the start on
a couple-centered approach to care. All a man need do is refuse to respond
to requests from the medical system—a common occurrence—or take another "fertile" wife for the entire treatment plan to fall upon the woman.

Though low sperm levels (oligospermia) or simply their absence (azo-
ospermia) might be revealed through medical testing, these diagnoses
may be deliberately concealed, according to some of my informants. Male
solidarity can shift responsibility once again to the woman. For example,
Madame HS1, like Madame HZ1, reported that she had long been alone in
taking charge of the couple's infertility. She recounts her marital drama:

> My husband was sterile. His sperm weren't viable (*nga haro a sinda amfani* [Z];
> literally, "his water was worthless"). But I was practically the last person to know
> after undergoing many treatments myself. I was subjected to exams and even
> minor surgeries for two and a half years with no success. I went to follow-up
> visits and examinations with other specialists who found my body and my *haytu*
> (uterus) healthy and normal. That was when I asked my husband to also have
> a routine exam (spermogram). He went to the doctors I'd seen first, some of
> whom were friends of his. They detected the problem but secretly prescribed
> medication to combat his condition, which is said to have a 60% chance of being
> treated. They told me he was in good health. Which I believed for a while. After
> six months, I happened to find a leaflet in the trash for the drugs he was taking
> regularly. That was when I realized I'd been tricked all along. I took the leaflet
> to multiple people to understand it. It's obvious! My husband produced weak
> sperm. Even though it took a long time—18 months—for him to admit it and
> to apologize. The damage is done. It's too late. I went home to my parents and
> quickly asked for a divorce. This man has destroyed my life. Because of my al-
> leged sterility, his family has never been kind to me, not even his friends, who

have often been very rude. I've seen people come sit in our living room to wait for my husband and not bother to say "hello" or "good evening" to me. Now that I'm clear of all suspicion, they want me to stay with him so as not to tarnish his reputation. Everyone, starting with my family and his, have gotten involved to stop the separation. I've tried everything, with no success. I know what I have to do now . . . [silence, followed by a long sigh] get this divorce paper [certificate of divorce]. I have to start my life over. I'm only 28 years old. It's not too late to have children. (Madame HS1, 28 years old, teacher, companion of a woman giving birth, Boukoki Maternity)

I interviewed this woman at the beginning of my study in 2003. When I met with her toward the end of this project, she had finally divorced but had not been able to remarry as quickly as she wanted. She had, however, become pregnant with twins in the meantime. The father, a man already in a polygamous marriage, had recognized the pregnancy. She told me that they planned to marry. This extra-marital pregnancy, despite being socially objectionable, is gradually being accepted by her friends and family. This illustrates how having children under conditions deemed deviant can be regarded as better than remaining childless. A marriage between Madame HS1 and the father of her children appears to be socially acceptable, particularly as twin pregnancies place women on a pedestal. "They call me 'tawey nya' ('the mother of twins' [Z])," she says with pride. It doesn't matter how these twins were conceived—they fill a void that society abhors.

Because it was not linked to erectile failure, the sterility of HS1's husband gave rise to various stratagems to clear him of any responsibility. It is certainly possible that adultery, when it meets the need for perpetuation of the group and conceals the physical and biological faults of men, takes on an almost institutional form. This solidarity around infertile men reveals the ideological prevalence of female responsibility in couples struggling with infertility.

By refusing to accompany their wives or to undergo treatment programs at their own initiative, many men (like the husbands of Madame HZ1 and Madame HS1) choose between two options that do not always favor their wives: repudiation or polygamy.

THEORETICAL CONTRIBUTIONS ON FEMALE RESPONSIBILITY

How can this concealment of male infertility be explained? In settings where marriage is the vehicle for the perpetuation of a lineage, the woman is considered to be the first in charge of fertility because procreation implicates the woman more heavily, while the sexual act is more or less committed by the man (Bouchard 2000). Binary social logic associates women with procreation, while sex is a purely male domain (André 1985).

Françoise Héritier noted that in many anthropological studies, particularly those written about patrilineal societies, sterility "is automatically understood as feminine" (1984: 125). In her research, Héritier emphasized that the high visibility of female failure to conceive presents an analytical problem. Anthropologists themselves neglect the existence of male sterility "not so much because the authors applied their own cultural assumptions to the data they collected, but because the data were formulated in this way by the informants themselves" (p. 130). She concludes that male sterility, aside from impotence, is not socially recognized. The problem arises because "if only women give birth to both sexes, thus claiming the exclusive privilege of fertility . . . it follows that in the same logic, sterility is also a female prerogative. If women who are normally fertile do not give birth, it is thought that the hostile femininity in them refuses it" (Héritier 1984: 125).

In a study of abortion among Yoruba women in Nigeria, Winny Koster notes that "Women are always the prime suspects when a couple cannot produce children; they are the indicators of fertility because they get pregnant and not the husband (although it is acknowledged that men can also be infertile)" (2003: 293). The lack of male responsibility in a couple's difficulty conceiving is also highlighted by Houda El Aaddouni in the largely Muslim Moroccan context: "sterility, knowledge of it, and its healing and treatment have traditionally been a woman's business. This business, transmitted from generation to generation, ensures continuity between the worlds of yesterday and today in the permanent tension of a trajectory into the future" (2003: 47). The accusations that women face for being infertile shed light on both the societal value placed on reproduction and the power of patriarchy.

Holding the woman responsible for a couple's infertility stretches beyond an African framework; it is almost universal. Mireille Laget noted that in pre-modern France as well, it was the woman who was considered responsible for sterility because she either did or did not carry the child: "we did not imagine that men can be incapable of procreating" (1982: 37). Even in relatively developed countries, women are the first to be examined. It is only once their "physiological normality" has been verified that we turn to men. Laurence Pourchez states, "Even if women are, in large part, aware of the possibility of male sterility, unspoken codes and social pressures, particularly from the husband's family who wishes to see the continuation of their lineage, ensure that focus is on the female causes of the couple's sterility" (2002: 63).

In reading the literature that addresses this question, it becomes clear that it is particularly difficult to engage male responsibility in a couple's infertility when the man does not suffer from erectile dysfunction. However, in light of data collected in the field, it is important to put Héritier's analyses (as well as those that share common threads) into perspective because male sterility is not entirely ignored. Here I am interested in the strategies used to hide it. Male infertility is generally overlooked until all other remedies have been exhausted. With the progress of medical technology, Héritier's universal claims have less relevance. As Madame HS1 and some of her peers insist, male infertility does exist even if society's manipulation of its own rules allows men more room to maneuver. Ultimately, the tremendous attention to female infertility is only equaled by the noisy silence regarding male infertility. The man is not suspected until a new wife (or wives) has entered his home and suffered reproductive disappointment.

STERILITY SYMBOLISM

Like Koster, I found in my research a dialectic between representations of fertility and infertility "such that understanding one leads to a much greater understanding of the other" (2003: 261). In practice, it is difficult to talk about infertility without referring to fertility; they draw their meanings from each other.

The Fertile Earth, the Fertile Woman

Female reproductive virtues are surrounded by a host of symbolic representations. One of the most common—closely tied to the fertility of the earth—associates sexuality with food and the mouth with genitals in such a way that procreative and nourishing functions are interlaced. The equivalency of femininity and certain natural categories (plants, water, earth, etc.) is not exclusively African. These types of "cosmocentric" considerations drive the daily experience of ancient and contemporary peoples (Gélis 1984; Laget 1982; Gélis, Laget, and Morel 1978). It is generally accepted that the fertility of the earth is connected to female fertility. In many popular conceptions, the abundance of the harvest is thus intimately linked to the status of the mother-woman, who alone seems to know the mysteries of creation and the origin of life. In this symbolism of reproduction, she transmits her fertility to the earth, which in turn produces an abundant harvest. The same belief likens the woman to the field and the man to a dispenser of seed; the generative act is likened to plowing. From these analogies between the nutritive earth and the vital source-carrying woman, an inverse symbolic representation associates the infertile earth to the sterile woman. These are similarities that have been noted in many studies of African societies. Héritier's research draws connections between sterility, heat, drought, and aridity (1984). Bodo Ravololomanga (1992: 18) reports that the Malagasy also compare a sterile woman to "'dry, arid land' (*tanin gazana*) thus uncultivated and unproductive, which is contrary to the image of the nutritive earth she should embody." A male healer I interviewed develops a similar idea:

> The farmer whose wife doesn't conceive is a man who can't live from his harvest, because his wife's sterility is directly transmitted to the land. When your wife is sterile, your field always produces much less than those of others. She passes her misfortune to the soil, which is in turn struck with the inability to produce. . . . I swear, these are two things that are closely linked. You can't have one without the other. The man whose wife is fertile never fails: his business flourishes, his field is productive, all his endeavors are met with success. That's the way it is, madam! . . . Earth symbolizes the nourishing mother for every human being. In a way, it's from the earth that we're born; it's what feeds us. This too is reciprocal. Through our fertility, we make it possible for the earth to continue to support us. In death, it's she who receives us. Everything comes from the earth and returns to the earth. (HB, 47 years old, eight children, healer, Yantala district)

The idea of the reciprocity of influences between the earth and humans is prominent.

Ouassa Tiékoura, who analyzes the factors leading to Nigerien women's entry into prostitution, recalls that the childless wife enjoys no social recognition as she is compared to "land which one nourishes, but which remains unproductive—her fate is hardly enviable in a society where only her role as a producer of the workforce is valued" (1997: 348). She reminds us that, within agricultural systems, we commonly consider plants that do not reproduce as "male." All that relates to fertility is strictly linked to the feminine, whereas a contrary value is associated with the masculine. And in the same vein, Doris Bonnet (1988: 26) teaches us that "in Mossi society, everything that is male is symbolically associated with sterility." This gendered categorization of animal or plant beings is also omnipresent in Nigerien society.

Infertility as Social Death

Some of my interview subjects, like this traditional barber whose first wife has suffered from secondary infertility for nine years,[1] associate infertility with death:

> Our parents live through us. We always refer to their children as the achievements they've had on earth. In the same way, to show we really exist, we must have children in our turn, otherwise it's as if you don't exist. Whether you have a job, a good situation—in the eyes of others, all this is secondary compared to having children who represent the real effort we've made on earth. For example, the money you earn—you're not the one who produces it. A child, though, is your own creation—it's a part of you. So you can imagine how people who've never reproduced live—it's as if they've never existed; they're still incomplete. In a way, sterility is death. (YI, 49 years old, father of 11 children, traditional barber, Talladjé district)

Pierre Erny (1988: 327) notes that "the immortality awaited by the African man is realized less in his personal survival than in a kind of collective eternity, his presence perpetuated through progeny." The idea of bankruptcy also calls to mind an image close to death. Ravololomanga (1992: 77) signals that "the ideas of death and sterility are combined into one and the same calamitous concept—*manjo*—which means misfortune and mourning."

Failed immortality caused by the absence of children often justifies the pity expressed toward sterile individuals. Yet, this pity is accompanied by condemnation. Most analyses of agricultural societies, whether socio-anthropological (Héritier 1978, 1984, 1996, 2002; Erny 1988; Lacoste-Dujardin [1985] 1996; Koster 2003), historical (Gélis 1984; Laget 1982; Bologne 1988), or demographic (Locoh 1984, 1991; Caldwell 1982; Caldwell and Caldwell 1987) agree on the convergence of feelings of permanent commiseration and strong stigmatization to which childless women are subjected in their daily lives. The sterile woman is considered guilty and

---

1. According to medical terminology, "primary infertility" applies to a person who has never had a child, while "secondary infertility" occurs after at least one conception.

solely responsible for her lamentable situation. Infertility hinders the woman's other, no less important, role in society: that of production. Unable to supply children—a source of filial ties and a force of production—she is therefore doubly useless to society.

Infertile, Therefore a Witch

Witchcraft, which is omnipresent in sub-Saharan Africa, is regularly linked to sterility. It will be noted that witchcraft is evoked in two different ways in the popular beliefs documented in my research. A sterile woman may be accused of carrying the seeds of witchcraft within her. In Niamey, this type of thinking is mainly found among people from other countries in the sub-region. Women of Togolese, Beninese, and Ivorian nationality who were included in this research indicated witchcraft as the origin of sterility, using the French term *sorcière*: "A witch cannot give birth to a child. Her wickedness doesn't allow it" (Madame KM, 33 years old, mother of four children, shopkeeper, Nouveau Marché district).

Among these populations' mystical belief systems, sterility stems from the devouring actions of a woman who eats her offspring before birth. This "devouring mother" is somewhat different from the one described by Denise Paulme (1986) because here the children are annihilated before they even see the light of day.[2] A woman's malice, then, can be the cause of her sterility. Wickedness is the main component of the "witch's" identity, and it is believed that she consciously refuses to make the distinction between a part of herself (her child) and others. The causal link between witchcraft and infertility implies that one is infertile because one is a witch. As HB, a 47-year-old healer with eight children told me, "It's very common that a *cerkow* [(Z) sorceress] woman can't have children." When a malicious inner force animates the infertile person, all signs of life, it seems, distance themselves from her.

According to Ravololomanga (1992: 80), the sterile woman in Madagascar is characterized by bitterness and asocial tendencies and appears, in the eyes of others, as a witch. Bonnet makes the same observation among the

---

2. Some tales and legends from West Africa recorded by Paulme show that the fear of being suffocated by motherhood can push a mother to swallow her children. This devouring mother "ignores the essential feminine function—transmitting life—and acts inversely, swallowing humans, domestic animals, and all the evidence of a creative presence that she finds on her way. The mother no longer gives birth, she devours" (1986: 286). The mythical figure of the mother is always fluid as it combines both the image of the nurturing mother and that of the greedy mother, bearer of death.

Mossi, where the sterile person is considered misfortunate, a woman abandoned by her ancestors. In that setting accusations of what Bonnet calls "symbolic anthropophagy" are mainly brought against women (1988: 72). According to some studies, witchcraft can take unique forms due to the socially institutionalized circulation of children. Younger women, presumed to resent the confiscation of their offspring for the benefit of older women, may be suspected of witchcraft if the child dies (Bonnet 1988: 104).

Infertility and Masculinity

> It's the fact of carrying a child for several months that defines a woman. When a woman has never had this experience, she has the appearance of a man. (HB, 47 years old, eight children, healer, Yantala district)

As this interviewee maintains, and as did many others after him, femininity is achieved through motherhood. Many popular beliefs, not simply in Niger, present the infertile woman as an incomplete person who experiences a "failure of identity" because fertility is viewed as central to the identity of women (Fine 2002: 67). In some discourses it is posited that she is not, strictly speaking, a woman: "Whether positive or negative, failed woman or failed man, she is closer to the man than to the woman. Thus, it is not sex but fertility which defines the real difference between masculine and feminine" (Héritier 1996: 230). The social tendency to associate infertile women with the male body is very important. This denial of femininity from women who have never conceived is a challenge to their gender identity.

> Some people think that what makes the difference between a man and a woman is the pregnant body. When a woman has never been pregnant, she's not far from a man. My co-wife was mean enough to say that to me one day. This is exactly what she said: "*nin nda alboro kulu afo day no ay diyon ga*" ([Z] literally, "in my opinion, you're the same as a man"). (Madame ZI, 33 years old, childless, woman operated on at the Central Maternity Hospital)

POPULAR SEMIOLOGY OF STERILITY

The Hausa and Zarma languages spoken by a large majority of my interviewees are rich with regard to questions of fertility and infertility. The rejection of sterile women has produced semantics that are pejorative, satirical, and stigmatizing. The different local languages are largely silent on male sterility.

The concealment of male sterility is socially shared. The semantics of female sterility are based heavily on the stomach, which is the receptacle of the child and thus the receptacle of life.[3] For men, reference is made to the penis which, by secreting seminal fluid, is the true provider of life. The expressions used are generally experienced as humiliating by the people to whom they are addressed. This derogatory lexicon is often used during arguments or fights intended to be offensive. The pity that is generally felt toward a sterile woman can develop into persecution. Pejorative expressions are mainly used by women (co-wives, sisters-in-law, etc.) and, to some extent, by the husbands of sterile women. In these cases, the man's objective is often to create conditions for the spontaneous departure of his wife from the marital home when he has not been able to obtain this result by other means.[4] It must be said that some women, despite their husbands' attempts at repudiation or divorce, continue to hold onto a married life that has turned its back on them.

In Zarma, the commonly used term to designate a sterile person is *gunu*.[5] The sterile woman is said to be *way-gunu*. Here, the semiology has no particular connotation: this phrase is neither pejorative nor favorable. In Hausa, the onomatopoeic *kararia* conveys the idea of emptiness. The semantic origin of this term is difficult to determine. According to some of my interviewees, it could be related to the Arabic term *âquera*, which is also used to designate a sterile woman in the Islamic tradition; I am unable to confirm this theory.[6]

Jokes made in poor taste, dark humor, and other jibes are often used to deride a sterile person. One of the rare expressions linked to male sterility incorporates the impotent penis in the parody of sterility. The Zarma expression *alboro kan bu* means "a dead man" and refers to an impotent man whose penis has no erectile capacity. The expression specifically refers to the dead, inactive penis. A simple extrapolation of the "dead penis" and the biological impossibility of having children echoes the kind of social death described above.

3. Editor's note: In Hausa the word *ciki* means "inside" as well as "stomach" and "womb."

4. Editor's note: When a marriage is dissolved at the initiative of the wife, her family must return the bridewealth that formalized the marriage to the husband. If he unilaterally repudiates her, the bridewealth is her family's to keep. Husbands therefore attempt to provoke their spouses to leave, while wives' families encourage them to go back.

5. *Gunu*, used as a noun and pronounced differently, also designates one who circumcises. It can also be a type of Songhai magician (Olivier de Sardan 1982: 174).

6. Chebel (2004), who reports the names used to designate sterile women in the Maghreb, notes that, depending on the regions and local phonetics, the terms *âkera* or *aguerra* might apply.

A sterile man or woman, considered responsible for their own condition, may be exhorted to try harder. Through a logic of imputation, critics incriminate a sterile person's will without ever raising the question of physical or physiological problems. Madame HS2, a woman without children, thus attributes these words to her detractors: "You're sterile because you wanted to be, you could be fertile if you wanted to." This opinion prevails in public discourse. Rather than registering victimization, this manner of speaking attributes guilt. The belief is that the origin of sterility lies in an internal opposition between the individual and the forces of life.[7]

If we buy into this logic, the accused person could, by force of their own will, work to resolve this challenge. Increasingly, certain so-called progressive women, notably civil servants and some educated women, are criticized for wanting to adopt "a White life" that is less suited to a family life centered around offspring. This is a life based on the Western model in which fewer children are desired. This criticism is made when the birth of the first child is delayed or when much time passes between two births. Sometimes accusers denounce the postponement of motherhood or an "unreasonable" spacing between births, rather than the outright renunciation of motherhood, which, as I have described above, is presumed to not be possible. It is only when the woman is too old to have children that this idea is finally abandoned, and then we look to other causes for the absence of children.

Woyboro kan go ga nwa ga maani margu is a common Zarma expression that means literally "a woman who does nothing but eat to fatten herself." In other words, the stomach of the woman in question is only used for digesting food when, necessarily, it should house and produce a child. By becoming a simple receptacle for food, a woman's stomach signals her social uselessness. A woman's round pregnant stomach is viewed as bestowing upon her the glory attained through motherhood.

A similar Hausa expression, *ciki ka yi daaji*, translates as "stomach used for defecation." The symbolism of the stomach in the Nigerien context refers to both the processes of consumption and of childbirth. The allusion that is made to food whenever a woman is sterile creates a hierarchy between the two events. Giving birth comes before the need for food. "What's the use of continuing to eat when you're alone in the world, with no children?," as one

7. From a psychological and psychoanalytic approach, Deutsch has shown that psychological causes can disturb the physiological process and lead to sterility in women: "Considered a functional disorder, infertility of psychic origin in women is a very complex and stubborn phenomenon; its root cause is generally difficult to uncover, even when modern methods of investigation can reveal hormonal disturbances" ([1949] 1987: 95).

of my respondents said as an aside. Another woman complained of her son's futile efforts (*a go ga taabi* [Z]) to provide food for his wife, though she does nothing to have a child and logically should one day repay the material and mystical investments which have been made on her behalf.

Men are less severe toward other men who do not manage to produce descendants than women are toward one another. A review of popular semiology shows that women are not very tolerant of infertile women. Sisters, sisters-in-law, and cousins most often have ambiguous, competitive, and potentially conflictual relationships. They never fail to remind one another of their flaws when they see fit.

EMIC INTERPRETATIONS OF STERILITY

The quest for meaning and causation has always been at the base of popular interpretative systems. Like a sick person, the sterile woman lives a misfortune linked to an external cause. As Nicole Sindzingre writes, "Being the subject of misfortune is fundamentally unfair for anyone, and involves the need to find meaning, to insert the event into a chain of causation and effects—to find an explanation" (1984: 96). In West Africa, there is a language of evil and a symbolic logic that surrounds the social perception of sterility and many other maladies (Olivier de Sardan 1999b). The naming of a disease gives meaning to its symptoms, while putting an end to the quest for meaning; this is the *logic of designation*. Diseases that cannot be named are identified instead by the presumed responsible agent. In this case, we enter a *logic of imputation*. For some who subscribe to the logic of designation, sterility is a natural disease that can be curable provided the correct remedy is found. For those who attribute it to a supernatural force, the etiology of sterility can only be magico-religious:

> If someone cast a spell on you to not have children, as is often the case between co-wives, you have to reach out to the marabouts and traditional healers if you hope to be healed. (Madame TS, 61 years old, traditional healer, Gamkallé district)

Whether it is a man or a woman who struggles to conceive children, the search for meaning is quite often part of the search for treatment. The interpretations assigned to sterility range from the man's impotence (also designated by the expression "dead penis") to transgenerational conflicts and include amenorrhea, blood incompatibility, sexual transgressions, witchcraft, and the myth of the sleeping child. Some explanations overlap. The forbidden acts of incest and adultery, for example, are closely linked to the idea of divine and social sanction, just as impotence and amenorrhea are for their part sometimes attributed to the enigmatic laws of fate.

BODILY IMPEDIMENTS TO CONCEPTION

The Man with the "Dead Penis"

Impotence, the male manifestation of sterility, is absent from the discourse on this subject. The inability of a man to have an erection is a pathology that does exist, but it is probably uncommon. It is difficult to say whether the rarity of this occurrence is genuine or whether impotence simply benefits from social reticence. While in women biological motherhood is identified by its physical aspects, by its palpable characteristics, biological paternity in men, supported by a "semantic restriction" (one cannot grasp the sentence "he gave birth") is much more difficult to delineate. Indeed, the sacred principles of motherhood and fatherhood on which all pronatal societies are based obligate women and men to fulfill their respective mission in the perpetuation of society unconditionally. However, socially determined paternity can benefit sterile men.

As a general rule, "impotent" men are not able to maintain a stable married life. Women who have been married to such men leave soon after the wedding week or a few months later.

> Attempts to hide such an affliction are usually unsuccessful. (MN, 54 years old, seller of aphrodisiac products, Talladjé district)
> When a man's penis doesn't work, when he has a dead penis, no woman can stay long. If he marries a young girl who doesn't know anything about men, he can keep her until she understands these things. It's not easy with the girls in Niamey. (A traditional healer)

Complete Amenorrhea

One could say that amenorrhea (the absence of menstruation) is the female counterpart of impotence (Héritier 1984).[8] It is generally considered

8. The medical system generally distinguishes between two types of amenorrhea: primary amenorrhea and secondary amenorrhea. Both are characterized by the absence of menstruation. The first is due to pre-pubescent age (often before 13 years of age). The second occurs when a woman who has previously menstruated sees her periods disappear for at least three months. Secondary amenorrhea is a "condition" most common in postmenopausal women. By "complete amenorrhea" I mean the total absence of menstruation, located at the extreme of each of these two main forms.

the most extreme case of female infertility. Amenorrheic women experience sterility. In the popular imagination of the Samo of Burkina Faso, it results in an overflow of heat, which these women accumulate and are never able to evacuate (Héritier 1984). In these cases, it is neither prepubescent amenorrhea nor contraceptive or menopausal amenorrhea. It is a disorder resulting in the complete absence of menstruation. Women of reproductive age who experience amenorrhea occupy a position of "maximal abnormality" with respect to female identity. If conception is the most determining and constitutive element of female identity, menstruation is also a marker of femininity: menstruation and breasts are the primary attributes of femininity which converge toward motherhood.

> The minimum that can be required of a normal young woman is her period. Otherwise, there's nothing feminine about her. We can't even identify her as a man, because they secrete the water that makes the child.[9] She's not like women or men. (YI, 49 years old, father of 11 children, traditional barber, Talladjé district)

The absence of menstruation is even more stigmatized than sterility itself. It leads to double stigmatization—that facing the woman without menstruation and that facing the woman without a child. Unlike some women who believe in blood incompatibility and cling to the hope of pregnancy with a different partner, women without menstruation have no illusion of future motherhood.

> I have never had a period. I'm over forty now. When I consulted healers, I always asked them to make my period come first since you can't hope to become pregnant without a period. Because I never had them, I never harbored false hopes of having children. (Madame DD, 43 years old, childless, housewife, Dar-Es-Salam district)

Yet, some belief systems consider these women to be individuals whose destiny has been chosen by God. Through them, God's celestial force is made visible. Unlike cases in which sterility is considered as the consequence of a sanction, it is in some settings perceived as a form of divine grace. In these rare contexts, women can positively reappropriate amenorrhea, even while keeping their lack of menstruation hidden. In Niger such women may be designated by the generic expression *annabi woyey* (Z), whose literal

---

9. "Water" refers here to seminal fluid.

meaning is "wives of the Prophet."[10] During my research I only encountered two non-menstruating women, aged 29 and 43 years, respectively. The first underwent a few treatments at health centers but said that she gave up on it quickly for lack of results. Both think of themselves as *annabi woyey* and have become invested in mastering Islamic culture by memorizing verses from the Qur'an. The older, having memorized the entire Qur'an, is already a scholar, while the younger also said that she was on her way to becoming accepted as a scholar.[11]

Blood Incompatibility: Shared Responsibility

In the local traditional therapeutic system, sometimes an incompatibility of sexual partners is linked to a clashing of bloods or of the man's seminal fluid with the woman's body. This is commonly called "blood incompatibility," which is believed to stem from the inability of two spouses' blood to fuse during sexual intercourse. It is said that the bloods refuse to commingle, thus blocking any possibility of fertilization. In medical spheres, this may be an incompatibility between the sperm and the vaginal environment. There is also talk of difficulty in finding "harmony" between the woman's ovum and the man's sperm. Overall, blood incompatibility can be translated into local languages as *kuray si saba* (Z) and *rishin jituwan jini* (H). In these cases, each spouse must make a new life with another partner. According to this interpretation of infertility, both spouses are exonerated.

> When there is blood incompatibility between a man and his wife, they are forced to separate. Each must marry another partner. (MN, 54 years old, seller of aphrodisiac products, Talladjé district)

As Héritier's study found among the Samo, I found that such spouses may choose either to separate or to stay together. In the latter case, the man must enter a second marriage to bring the benefit of children to his household that he has failed to achieve with his first wife. The first wife thus commits herself "voluntarily" to a childless existence. In extreme cases,

10. These considerations are especially prevalent in rural areas. In their Zarma–French dictionary, however, Bernard and White-Kaba (1994: 305) emphasize that the expression *annabi way* (*way* or *wey* is the singular of *woyey*) is used to designate a "woman with very small breasts."

11. The proscription of handling the Qur'an, praying, or performing pilgrimage while menstruating makes a life devoted to Islamic learning difficult for women before they enter menopause. The absence of menstruation favors devotional practice.

some couples who have suspected this type of problem have tried their luck separately in extra-marital affairs while maintaining their bonds of marriage. The socially deviant nature of this type of conduct effectively creates the conditions for its concealment and censorship in speech as well as in conduct. Although rare in my research, the notion of blood incompatibility as an interpretation for sterility seems to restore a certain balance between the sexes.

ACTS OF SEXUAL TRANSGRESSION THAT THREATEN FERTILITY

Sterility is also associated with certain transgressions. Among these offenses are sex out of wedlock, crimes of adultery, and incestuous sex. Elsewhere, as in Gouro society in Côte d'Ivoire, having sex during menstruation may be understood to cause female sterility (Haxaire 2003); but that is not the case in Niamey. Many of my respondents believe, rather, that copulation with a menstruating woman may provoke various disorders in men, including sexually transmitted diseases or even impotence.

Pre-marital Sexuality

Pre-marital sex is one explanation offered for infertility in women. This infertility is experienced by the guilty person as a form of punishment. Contrary to biomedical interpretations, where reproductive dysfunction is often attributed to sexually transmitted diseases (interpretations that are accepted by local government, educated individuals, and other "progressives"), infertility is evoked much more commonly as punishment for a moral transgression in emic conceptions.

> Having sex before the prescribed time—marriage—has serious consequences, like staying sterile. It's a form of punishment. (Madame Hadjia A, 52 years old, companion of a patient undergoing an operation)

Koster underscores the sense in Yoruba society in Nigeria that it may be better to have illegitimate children than to go childless altogether (2003: 89). Here, too, in some circles, despite the social stigma of a birth out of wedlock, non-birth remains the ultimate curse. The aggression and reproaches of a woman's social circle (parents, acquaintances, friends, and allies) during the first months of pregnancy may give way to tenderness toward the fatherless child. Similarly, there are examples of women who have experienced one or more pregnancies out of wedlock during their adolescence who have been able to settle into a stable married life and free themselves from their image of a depraved young girl. The children who they birthed with their husbands served to erase their "bad girl" image, and they have managed to gain respectability (see the story of Madame HS1 above). This is the retrospective wish of a 43-year-old woman who had a child out of wedlock who died at the age of 13. She has struggled to conceive with her husband for the last 15 years:

> I would've liked to have had several children without a father. I regret having only had one. I would've also liked him to survive—he alone would have made me happy, even if one child is very little. (Madame IM, 43 years old, childless, Balafon district)

This is proof that, beyond prescribed social norms, it is easier to forgive the young woman who is found to no longer be a virgin on her wedding night and the young girl who behaved badly by having illegitimate children than it is to forgive the sterile woman. Similarly, Tiékoura (1997) links some women's recourse to prostitution in Niamey with the desire for maternity. To these women, promiscuity may be a last resort to access maternity. For these women the ends justify the means. These seemingly deviant behaviors (including adultery, which I discuss below) place the apparent rigidity of social norms and the notion of unconditional submission to such norms in perspective. Such contradictions and inconsistencies render the binary analysis of right and wrong moot.

Extra-Marital Sex: Adulterous Practices

> God doesn't forgive fornicators of any kind, but even less when they're held to the sacred rules of marriage. God dries up any woman who cheats on her husband. She doesn't deserve to have a child. God will curse her and take the joy of being a mother away from her. (Malam I, 44 years old, marabout-healer, Boukoki district)

Women guilty of pre-marital sexual debauchery are generally considered "sexual nomads." But we will also see that some women turn to adultery in the hope of providing their sterile home with children. According to one traditional healer, if a woman has multiple sexual partners, "the mixture of sperm from different origins" corrupts the quality and prevents conception.

Some women go from one man to another before marriage. These are the same women who, once married, can't be satisfied by their husbands. They'll always look elsewhere. In these conditions, how do you expect them to receive the divine blessing of children? God punishes them for their delinquency. (AH, 45 years old, traditional healer, Boukoki district)

Pre- or extra-marital sexuality, however, can indeed lead to pregnancy, which in some cases is quickly terminated. Luc Boltanski, in his sociological study of the generalized taboo on abortion even where legal, observes that sanctions for such transgressions "are either immanent to the act itself (such as sterility) or diffuse penalties that affect the kinship group or even the collective body as a whole (for example, in the wake of an act of vengeance carried out by the spirit of the aborted foetus), as is often the case when transgressive practices affect the order of the world" ([2004] 2013: 16). This logic also prevails in Niger. A close link is made between sexual acts and deviant abortions leading to the punishment of primary or secondary infertility.

Incestuous Sexuality

The prohibition of incest is a universal phenomenon even if the forms it takes vary from one society or culture to another. Evans-Pritchard (1951: 30) offers a classic description of incest:

> When it is forbidden for a man to have relations with a woman he may not, of course, marry her, and it will be simpler to begin this account by stating the Nuer table of marriage prohibitions. Marriage is not permitted between clansfolk, close cognates, close natural kinsfolk, close kinsfolk by adoption, close affines, and persons who stand to one another as fathers and daughters in the age-set system.

For both men and women, in Niger, respecting the prohibition of incest protects one from sterility.

> A father who sleeps with his daughter or a mother who has sex with one of her sons commits the vilest act of one's whole life. In my opinion, it would be better for a mother to kill her child than to sleep with him. Eh . . . neither ties of blood nor milk can forgive that. Bad luck will come to all parties in their turn. For those who do not yet have children, sterility is the punishment that most commonly awaits them. (A woman at a family planning consultation session at an integrated health center, or *centre de santé intégré*, Talladjé district)

In Malagasy society, incest is believed to cause sterility (Ravololomanga 1992: 80). Similarly, in the Nigerien context any licentious relationship between two people linked by close family relationships, particularly between ascendants and descendants, at some point in their lives may cause sterility.

> A lot of people think the caretaker here slept with his daughter for a long time. He's had no other children since. Neither has his daughter, ever since she married. God punished them both. What an abomination! Even listening to this kind of story does harm, you might end up the same. May God keep us from such a fate! (Hadjia A, 52 years old, companion of a woman undergoing an operation)

This is less a divine punishment than a social punishment linked to what is commonly called "the force of milk" and, to a certain extent, "the force of blood." Both are evoked in legends as destructive and ruthless toward incest transgressions. Thus, a kind of sacred trust or *amaana* (H and Z) exists between a maternal uncle and his niece: the force of the "milk" relationship dissuades both from becoming involved in an intimate relationship. Likewise, between brothers and sisters, the force of milk and/or that of blood means that a sexual partnership must not occur; otherwise, the violation of *amaana* can strike one or both with sterility. Of the offenders, it will be said that the "*amaana* caught them" (*amaana a ni di* [Z] and *amaana ta kama su* [H]). For Olivier de Sardan (1982: 33), "The *amaana* has a sacred significance. To betray it is to automatically attract misfortune."

"OCCULT" PRACTICES THAT THWART FERTILITY

In many cases, infertility is attributed to malicious practices of witchcraft (related to anthropophagy), to evil spells of black magic, and to the "evil eye." The last two emic categories are closely related and sometimes conflated. Witchcraft and black magic are essentially evil and generally have a nefarious intent. In early modern Europe, medical texts ascribed infertility to magic or witchcraft (Bologne 1988: 58). Similarly, in contemporary Réunion, an infertile woman, "whose sterility could not be overcome by any means, who is an anomaly of nature, is suspected of wanting to harm fertile wives out of jealousy" (Pourchez 2002: 91). I will examine witchcraft, black magic, the "evil eye," and alliances with spirits as the main forms of "occult" practices understood to lead to sterility in Niamey.

Witchcraft, or *Carkowtaray*

Witchcraft in its true sense involves the seeking of aid from supernatural and potentially dangerous powers. For Olivier de Sardan (1982: 86), a *cerkow* is a sorcerer or witch who "steals men's 'doubles' (*biya* [Z]) to feed on them. The sorcerer can be a human, like you or me, who sometimes—especially in the evening—flees, turns into an animal (bird, headless donkey) and terrorizes people who are alone." In local semiology, witchcraft entails anthropophagy. "Soul eaters" (called *cerkow* [Z] and *maayu* [H]) can undermine a person's reproductive success.

> A *cerkow* is an evil being whose power reaches everywhere. It can kill a living person but can also prevent a child from being born by taking harmful action. (HB, 47 years old, eight children, healer, Yantala district)
>
> If a woman is in the grip of a *cerkow*, she can never give birth to a child. She can get pregnant but can never give birth to a living child. (YM, 31 years old, herbalist, Gamkallé district)

Black Magic

Magic considered "black" works differently. While the sorcerer personally attacks their victim, a specialist figure mediates between the victim and the sponsor of the dark magic. A "witch doctor" (*boka* [H] or *zimma* [Z]) calls upon their magic charms at the request of a client who wishes to harm someone.

A magical act aimed at a person's fertility generally draws its power from the spirit of revenge and corruption. Revenge can be sought by a co-wife, an unsuccessful suitor, a former spouse, or anyone who has a clear or latent rivalry. The co-wife and the rejected suitor (or former spouse) carry the seeds of vengeance within themselves. To appease this vengeance, they "tie up" their target by resorting to magic charms called *kotte* or *aleesi* (Z).[12] This action aims for the "symbolic closure" of the reproductive body. It is a kind of obstacle intended to thwart procreation. Unlike contraceptive knots (called *hawari* [Z]), this type of knot is made to permanently and involuntarily

---

12. The *kotte* plays a double role, both protective and malign. For Olivier de Sardan (1984: 259), "the *kotte* is at the center of individual and collective symbolic life; as the principal form of magical practices, it conveys each individual's hopes, fantasies, and fears." This charm can take any form: "It can be a simple spell (*jindiize*), an object (*kanji*) that one carries with them, a mixture that one ingests (like the millet cake *kusu*, named after the pot in which it is prepared)."

annihilate all chances of a woman's conception. The *kotte* is believed to act on the placenta of the woman, who is to remain permanently "tied."

> Our neighbor already had one child with her first husband. But since she's been in her new home—it must be four or five years now—she hasn't gotten pregnant. *Irkoy beeri*! (God is great! [Z]) Her co-wife seems determined to keep her from having children. At the Central Maternity Hospital, they tell her nothing's wrong with her; they say nothing's wrong with her husband, either. (Madame ZY, 29 years old, housewife, Lazaret district)

> Everyone knows H was "tied" by her former suitor. He doesn't want her to give a child to someone else. He was so mad; he'd spent his fortune on her and her family. And she left him for this other man at the last minute.[13] Today, she reaps the consequences. (Madame MN, 54 years old, seller of aphrodisiac products and housewife, Talladjé district)

While in Zarma *kotte* designates broadly everything related to black magic, in Hausa the term *dan baka* refers specifically to a charm that is cast to act negatively on a couple's reproductive life. Another Hausa charm, the *darmun gado*, serves to symbolically "tie" the bed of a married couple to avoid any fertilization in the marriage. No sexual relations between the couple will be fruitful.

The "Evil Eye"

Informants repeatedly referred to the evil eye as the source of infertility for certain women. This concept, synonymous with "jealousy," exists in both Hausa and Zarma. Whenever we are jealous and envious of someone or something, the way we look at them is necessarily malicious. Here, it is less of a question of magic or mystical force that we mobilize to harm our rival than the malice we spontaneously express. Speech joins with the gaze to attack the subject of envy with combined and recurrent force. For this reason, the mouth is generally used to illustrate the expression of this jealousy in emic conceptions. Victims are said to be affected by the mouth (*me* [Z]), tongue/language (*deene* [Z]), the "mouth of the world" (*baakin duniya* [H]), or the "evil eye" or the "malicious look" (*mo laalo* [Z]). Here, the "evil eye" has the

---

13. Editor's note: The process of courting a potential bride entails many gifts from the groom to his intended and her family. If she chooses not to marry him in the end, he is unlikely to get those gifts back.

same meaning as the "evil mouth." Among my interviewees, to "regard badly" and to "speak ill" produced the same occult and harmful consequences.

> We keep the beginning of a pregnancy secret as a precaution because we're too afraid of baakin duniya (worldly talk [H]). If someone makes a nasty remark about the pregnancy, there's a good chance the baby won't make it. It has nothing to do with maita (anthropophagia [H]), but it's very dangerous. If, for example, someone is bold enough to say "that belly is big," it's more than enough to trigger a miscarriage in the next hours or days. (Madame MN, 54 years old, saleswoman of aphrodisiac products, Talladjé district)

The "evil eye" or me/baakin duniya works when exercised abundantly: it requires excess to have effect. Indeed, talking too much about anything (a woman's pregnancy, a person's wealth or beauty, etc.) can have detrimental effects. If talked about enough, it will attract too much attention, and the subject of discussion will be struck with misfortune.

Alliances with Spirits

A woman may also remain infertile when possessed by a spirit who demands exclusive sexual relations with her. In such circumstances, a spirit may even oppose a girl's marriage when it becomes infatuated with her. The exceptionally long celibacy of some girls is often explained by this phenomenon. In extremely rare cases, the celibacy of certain men can also be linked to an alliance contracted with a water-dwelling female spirit. None of their romantic relationships result in marriage. Through a mysterious and repulsive force, the spirit-lover drives away all suitors or conditions the one possessed to refuse marriage.[14]

There is also the less extreme case of the spirit-spouse who accepts a woman's polyandry but who employs occult means to oppose the conception of a child. Any child conceived would be doomed from the start. It is often said that the spirit lives inside the woman's body, and her womb can no longer serve to shelter a child.

> We see people who can't conceive without any medically valid reason. But they're mainly women. When a woman isn't victim of kotte, it's surely because a spirit

---

14. Editor's note: Spirit possession cults can provide a socially recognized home for people whose gender identities and/or self-presentation defy the logic of heteronormative marriage and gender binaries.

lives in her or with her. In many cases, she can never get married. And when she's lucky enough to find a husband, she can't have children. (HB, 47 years old, eight children, healer, Yantala district)

Marabouts and healers generally focus on this as the potential cause of infertility during initial consultations with a woman in search of motherhood. The first question they ask women suffering from infertility is, "Do you often have sex in your dreams?" An affirmative response from the woman implies that a spirit has monopolized the exclusivity of the conjugal relationship, thus rendering impossible any hope of fertility for the legally married couple.

SUSPENDED FERTILITY: THE MYTH OF THE SLEEPING EMBRYO

People occasionally evoke the notion of "the sleeping embryo" to make sense of infertility. One woman I met during a medical consultation, Madame RT, was convinced that she has been pregnant for at least four years. She thought the progression of her pregnancy was suspended by some force such as those discussed above. A less occult understanding also exists in Islam; the "falling asleep" of the embryo may be understood to be of divine origins inaccessible to human understanding, an unresolvable mystery.

We see women who stay pregnant for almost ten years and then one day give birth. Others never give birth to the child they nevertheless carry. If she isn't using *hawari* [a form of contraception through charms made by a marabout or traditional diviner (Z)], it's difficult to explain a suspended pregnancy. (Alpha O., 50 years old, marabout-healer, Gaweye district)

A suspended pregnancy may more commonly be seen to result from malevolent magic, "tying the stomach," which leads to an either permanent or temporary "slumber" of the pregnancy. In the rare cases of a sleeping embryo, women believe that a happy ending is possible: the slumber will give way to a waking state, and the baby will be born. In this case, the child's "falling asleep" is linked to the *kotte* or the *dan baka* mentioned above, which is done without the woman's knowledge. The woman must be freed by breaking the enchantment with countercharms.

From the point of view of health professionals, this type of pregnancy is psychosomatic. In a final desperate impulse, but also in search of medical validation, Madame RT came in for an ultrasound to confirm her sleeping pregnancy, which ultimately revealed nothing. Healthcare providers explain that many of these women simply experience menstrual problems that are unrelated to pregnancy. While an abnormally long amenorrhea is sometimes assumed to indicate a pregnancy, other women who experience otherwise normal menstruation believe there is a "ball" in their stomach, which they take to be a developing child. Such a deduction on the part of these women can be easily understood: according to popular belief, a woman can in some cases carry a pregnancy while continuing to menstruate.

> In non-medical circles, people say a woman can have her period and be pregnant at the same time. It may just be minor bleeding due to physiological issues. But from there, they generalize and make people think the two can go together. This is why we've often seen women who claim to be pregnant while also reporting regular menstruation. (A caregiver at the Central Maternity Hospital)

As Madame RT's example shows, the popular classification of diseases is rarely consistent with that of the biomedical order. As Olivier de Sardan notes, "Never, anywhere, do popular representations of disease coincide with scholarly, biomedical representations" (1999a: 7). Madame RT's belief in her pregnancy has not been validated by the medical profession. The different descriptions that she tried to provide to the nursing staff suggest an "ambulatory logic" of a medical condition according to which something "circulates, moves, shifts, rises, descends" inside the human body (Olivier de Sardan 1999b: 77). Women who believe they are sheltering sleeping children also think that these often wander around in their wombs. While the logic of sleep and that of movement may seem glaringly contradictory, the two ideas combined make sense according to an ambulatory conception of illness. Lutz-Fuchs (1994) also reports on the myth of the "sleeping pregnancy" mentioned by some of his patients, who, however, unlike my interviewees, are mothers and may be in denial about entering menopause.

TRANSGENERATIONAL MISALIGNMENT

Typically, the right to sexual intercourse and procreation is exclusively held and appropriated by a single sexually active generation at a time (Héritier 1984). Bonnet notes that in Mossi society in Burkina Faso, "Some cases of infertility are interpreted as the consequence of a fertility that is 'monopolized,' so to speak, by some women of the lineage. So the capital is considered to be fairly (or unfairly) distributed among the different women of the lineage" (1988: 23). This implies that a young woman must wait for the decline of her mother's fertility to begin her sexual experience, while, conversely, the mother must end, if not her sex life, at least her "fertile career" at the moment her daughter crosses the threshold of the conjugal universe. Procreative forces pass from one generation to another, and the transfer takes place at the expense of the older generation. Occasionally in Niamey, informants invoked the principle that the pregnancy of a wife must coincide with the definitive renunciation of the procreative function of her mother but also of her mother-in-law. Transgenerational conflicts are thus almost inevitable. The social management of fertility imposes sexual and reproductive timelines on individuals. Just as there is an age to begin and end sexual activity, there is an age to begin and end reproductive life. The beginning of sexual and reproductive activity is part of the strict conjugal framework. It is paradoxically within this same socially legitimized framework that sexual relations and pregnancy may be castigated at a certain point:

> It's unacceptable to have pregnancies at the same time as the children you've given birth to. Honestly, it's not proper. A mother who continues to give birth when her married daughter is also of childbearing age does a lot of harm to the latter. Sometimes it's not forgiven and usually the daughter gives birth to only a few children or remains sterile. Here, the mother is so selfish that she took advantage of her own fertility and also got in the way of her daughter's. For the daughter to make her entry among mothers, her own mother must have already left her place among them. (OF, 40 years old, traditional healer from Mali, Maourey district)

This explanation for infertility, however, is not widespread in Niger. The question of generation and reproduction is more commonly referenced in the context of shame:

> A woman who knows shame avoids having children from the time her daughter gets married. Can you imagine this mother's daughter saying to her husband, "Mom had a baby" or "I'm going to my mother's baptism?" It's generally perceived as a great shame. The disgrace is shared by the woman and all those around her. (Madame HB1, 48 years old, eight children, Yantala district)

CONCLUSION

In this research I have been inspired by the theories of Françoise Héritier. Her work accords well with my own observations and conversations collected in the city of Niamey. Infertility is feminized. Only when the idea of "blood incompatibility" is advanced, which is rare, does infertility consider the relationship between a couple (considered as a unit) and not the individual (man or woman). The discourses surrounding the causes of infertility express "a homology of nature between the world, the individual body, and society, as well as the possibility of transfer from one of these registers to another. This homology is expressed with variable symbolic contents" (Héritier 1984: 24). According to various perspectives, witchcraft by a woman is a source of sterility. Because there is a natural order to the transmission of life force from one generation to the next, a mother's sexual and reproductive career must not overlap with her daughter's. Infertility is not seen as a physiological condition, even in cases of complete amenorrhea (Héritier 1984: 139).

Broadly, in the historical and anthropological literature, the misfortune of infertility is perceived to be the consequence of the past actions or behaviors of the suffering individual. Bologne suggests that in early modern Europe, "everyone is responsible for his own misfortune—whether the punishment is transcendent from a religious perspective or immanent from a medical perspective; guilt is the common denominator of all religions, including the scientism of the [nineteenth] century" (1988: 212). As found in my research, many studies on the phenomenon of sterility describe a similar logic of parsing out causation as due to divine, spiritual, or magical intervention (Rivière 1990; Ravololomanga 1992; Tichit 2009; Delaisi de Parseval and Janaud 1983; Gélis 1984; Flandrin 1984). The burden of responsibility, as we have seen, rests heavily upon women.

CHAPTER 2

Managing Infertility

Many of the subfertile women I encountered during my research emphasized their desperation and determination to have a child. The fight against infertility is constant, and the majority of women who suffer from it search ceaselessly for solutions, whatever the price to pay. The fears surrounding infertility have given rise to a multitude of practices, be they traditional, popular, or biomedical.[1] While some have a preventive function, others are curative. There are also methods that neither prevent nor treat the underlying causes of infertility but rather help concerned individuals and their relatives address the social problem of childlessness.

As I argue throughout this book, the management of human biological reproduction draws upon several interdependent spheres of social life: symbolic and social management by the family, biomedical interventions by trained medical personnel, and, quite prominently, the contributions of popular health practitioners. There is no coherent body of knowledge defining popular or traditional medicine. Popular specialists are consulted more commonly and are more trusted than biomedical specialists. The close relationships between healers and patients weigh considerably in favor of this sector. The biomedical system's vertical character is off-putting to many. Furthermore, popular therapies are often based on understandable homologies. In this chapter, I focus upon popular therapies to combat infertility.

---

1. Although itinerant sellers of pharmaceutical products appear to be relevant in infertility management elsewhere in West Africa (Haxaire 2003), none of my own informants said that they appealed to them for assistance in treating infertility.

Yearning and Refusal. Hadiza Moussa, Edited by Alice J. Kang and Barbara M. Cooper, Oxford University Press.
© Oxford University Press 2023. DOI: 10.1093/oso/9780197662113.003.0003

Unlike traditional and popular systems, the medical domain does not offer tools to prevent infertility beyond the prevention of contracting sexually transmitted diseases (STDs), one of the most common causes of infertility in both men and women. The discourse on the avoidance of STDs was disseminated initially to combat the AIDS pandemic, and it still provides little information on the implications of STDs for reproduction. Despite the significance of STDs as the principal cause of both primary and secondary infertility, the risk of becoming infertile due to these diseases is mentioned only tangentially in public health campaigns. Posters displayed inside health centers provide a fairly clear reminder of these risks. However, in broader public campaigns STD prevention is linked directly to avoiding human immunodeficiency virus (HIV)/AIDS rather than to the challenges with fertility that may follow. Perhaps out of shame, interviewees concerned about their subfertility who indicated that they have had premarital or extra-marital sexual activity discounted the impact of venereal diseases as a possible cause of their infertility.

Infertility has not traditionally been thought of as a public health problem, unlike the spread of HIV/AIDS, malaria, or rapid population growth. Internationally funded programs designed to promote birth control are ill suited to provide solutions for problems related to infertility, which are additionally quite expensive. For these reasons, infertility does not constitute a prominent public policy concern in Niger. Niamey, which boasts the country's first specialist center to address infertility concerns, does not have sufficient qualified personnel nor an adequate technical framework to meet demand. Oral remedies and surgical interventions remain the predominant methods of treatment. Moreover, in Niger's population policies, the focus lies entirely on decreasing fertility. The preoccupation with high fertility in Niger obscures the issue of infertility.

PREVENTATIVE METHODS

In many societies, the desire to ward off the specter of sterility has given rise to a variety of rites and practices, often magico-religious in character (Erny 1988; Gélis 1984; Koster 2003; Héritier 1984; Ravololomanga 1992; Rivière 1990). The yearning for children, and consequently the fear of childlessness, leads individuals down a range of paths of prevention. Often, the pharmacopeia is consulted first; certain herbs and plants are very popular. Expiatory or propitiatory sacrifices are also believed to combat infertility.

In the traditional sphere, the prevention of infertility takes place at two distinct levels. The first, as discussed in the preceding chapter, is based on a broad symbolism instantiated in incest prohibitions. But there are other prohibitions as well to ward off infertility. The second level employs various techniques combining traditional medicine with other therapeutic methods. These techniques are so culturally entrenched (so-called family recipes are the same preparations found within magico-religious circuits and vice versa) that it can be difficult to distinguish between traditional and popular remedies. These interdictions and techniques rest on a wealth of representations that are believed to varying degrees but broadly shared. During interviews these ideas were framed with phrases such as, "it can happen" or "it seems that it could be a result of."

Preventing Male Impotence

The prevention of male impotence is a prerequisite for the prevention of infertility. According to some popular conceptions, impotence can be avoided through one's attitude, manner, behavior, or comportment. Many of the prohibitions for men are closely linked to the inculcation of gender roles beginning at birth. These prohibitions serve to protect a man's virility, which is at risk when in contact with the world of women. The softness, weakness, and notorious fragility of the feminine domain can have a corrupting and defiling effect for boys and men. For example, young boys are forbidden from stepping over or sitting on a mortar or pestle because this would heighten the risk of their being sterile. This prohibition applies to all men, even adults, who are never immune to experiencing secondary infertility; even those who have proven their fertility by having children can lose their reproductive capacities.

Other taboos implicitly place the blame for male impotence upon the behavior of women. For example, one must never hit a boy with a kitchen spatula, for to do so is said to corrupt male virility. The preparation of the daily meal, made from a flour base (e.g., millet, sorghum, corn), requires a small spatula (*muccia* [H] or *kuru-bundu* [Z]) to work the dough (*tuwo* or *tuwon laushi* [H] or *kurba-kurba* [Z]). To correct an incorrigible and reckless child, one can imagine that an angry mother might use the first object she lays her hand on. The advice given to new mothers is to stay away from the kitchen during these moments of anger, far from these "devitalizing" utensils.

In the most common emic conceptions, milk, the primary nourishment for infants, is paradoxically perceived to be a potential cause of impaired virility in boys. It is thus emphatically forbidden for women to let their milk come into contact with their baby boy's genitals. If, despite all the precautions taken, this should happen, the mother is advised to quickly put a few drops of saliva on the "soiled" part, which is said to be able to counteract milk's damaging effects. I have observed this practice on numerous occasions. During medical consultations, I have seen women rush to wipe their children's genitals with saliva to neutralize the effect of milk accidentally dripped there. This was the case for Madame HS3, who was at a family planning consultation and hesitated before making the ritual gesture because the midwife had already talked to her on a previous occasion about the need for strict hygiene. She nonetheless completed the gesture under pressure from a person sitting next to her. Relieved, she said,

> I wanted to blow on his genitals quickly, but I was afraid of the midwife's reaction. You know that if I didn't do this, my child would never be a man. . . . Water isn't enough to destroy the effect of milk. You need your mother's saliva, because it was her mother's milk that caused the damage. (Madame HS3, 35 years old, three children, Gaweye district)

Interviewees also explained that certain foods deemed sexually devitalizing for men are to be avoided:

> Men should avoid eating sweet potatoes. It's a food reserved for women. The more a man eats them, the more he is sexually weakened. And the more he weakens, the less he's a man. In the long run, he risks not having children. (HB, 47 years old, eight children, healer, Yantala district)

Sexual failure can develop over time into reproductive weakness. The less a man shows sexual vitality, the less fertile he is. By contrast, cassava and its derivatives (gaari, tapioca) and dishes full of garlic and onions are highly prized for their stimulating and aphrodisiac properties. The same is true for honey.

Preventing Female Infertility

The prevention of infertility concerns both women and men. Social norms require that sexual intercourse take place preferably at night and out of sight of others and in particular forbid sex in the bush. The uncultivated bush is considered the home of ghosts, spirits, and evil natural forces. Because these invisible inhabitants occupy the bush, it would be too provocative to have intimate relations before their eyes. Human beings have no knowledge of their daily activities, and the reverse must also be true.

Other interpretations claim that, because they are invisible to the human eye, it is not uncommon for people to disturb resting spirits or to harm their children by trampling them, for example. Here, then, infertility takes the form of a mystical punishment whose resolution necessitates certain sacrifices.

Periods of bright moonlight are moments that bring beauty into people's lives, unlike times of total darkness, which is a source of danger and fear. For this reason, there is always a spike of activity on moonlit nights. Yet women and girls are advised against allowing the moon to "step over them." The moon's apparent course, from the moment of its appearance to its disappearance, has led to a belief that it moves. To stand in the moon's way, especially repeatedly, can therefore be a cause of infertility in women.

There are also rites of protection for pregnant women. They are part of a system to fight the onset of secondary infertility. To this end, the placenta is subject to a rather unique treatment. Great care is taken to bury the placenta to protect the mother from the risk of becoming sterile. This organ must neither fall into "evil hands" (*kamba laala* [Z]) nor be eaten by carnivorous animals. Some refuse to entrust its burial to women who have never given birth because such women might pass their infertility on to the new baby.

In the sphere of Islam, the prevention of sterility is also based on a number of prohibitions, particularly against sex outside of marriage. Unlike in the traditional sphere, where incest is seen as the most likely cause of infertility, Islam designates extra-marital sexual relations (adulterous, pre-marital for the unmarried, post-marital for the divorced or widowed) as blameworthy and inviting of the sanction of sterility. Fornication is considered an act of defilement for a Muslim. The rhetoric employed is meant to discourage any act of the flesh not legitimized by marriage.

> God is against fornication. Anyone who enters into sexual relations without being married is exposed to the punishment of God. (Malam I, 51 years old, marabout, Bagdad district)

The marabout exhorts Muslims to refrain from fornication and adultery to prevent infertility.

TREATING INFERTILITY

Because the desire for a child takes precedence over all other aspirations, women take fate into their own hands and deploy physical, psychological, symbolic, and material resources to satisfy it. The high stakes surrounding motherhood explain both the measures women take to treat infertility and efforts to prevent the premature death of their children. The tendency to employ multiple therapeutic remedies—sometimes in combination with one another—is fairly widespread. The range of anti-infertility cures is quite extensive, but it is difficult to measure their effectiveness.

This broad treatment system includes magico-religious practices and medical care through a multitude of techniques and procedures. Tunisian sociologist Abdelwahab Bouhdiba observes that "there is practically no institutionalized social role assigned to women other than that of mother. Hence the search for motherhood at all costs and the importance assumed by magico-religious practices and traditional medicines, a good part of which are oriented toward the fight against sterility and the increase of reproductive capacity" (2001: 265).

The many practices deployed to combat infertility in popular care settings are generally esoteric in nature and hidden from the non-practitioner. The treatments will vary by practitioner, and the methods can change over time. With no claim to exhaustiveness, I will present the remedies that marabouts and healers have been kind enough to share with me, as well as those cited by patients and their relatives. Because of the social invisibility of male infertility in Niamey, my outline of treatments for infertility focuses on those for female infertility.

Marabouts: Muslim Specialists

Muslim values constitute the basic spiritual frame of reference for most individuals in Niger. Maraboutic circles have gained legitimacy amid the "Islamic renewal" that has swept across Niger since the 1990s. While most Salafi Muslim preachers condemn divination and the use of charms in their sermons, the use of long-standing maraboutic remedies has increased. Marabouts, like other popular healthcare specialists, are in great demand in large urban centers like Niamey by both men and women. With talismans and various other maraboutic charms, men and women attempt to protect themselves or exorcise evils. People visit marabouts to pursue a number of ends: to facilitate professional promotion, for political advancement, or to solve marital problems, most commonly for the latter.

It is difficult to quantitatively document what could be called the solicitation of the occult, but it is clear that marabouts have not been excluded from the therapeutic market by Islamic reformers and that modern media can be leveraged to attract a large clientele. Certain "learned scholars" increasingly use the radio, print media, and cell phones to this end. Since the democratization movement in the 1990s, there has been a remarkable increase in private radio stations in Niamey. Private radio antennae are now widely used by marabouts renowned for their adept marketing of a broad range of new treatments for common contemporary conditions such as cancer, impotence, jaundice, infertility, and various STDs. The conditions "targeted" by these healers are those that feed anxieties and create a deep imbalance in the relationship between an individual and society as a whole. The pursuit of treatment for these conditions reveals the limits of medical science for Nigeriens. Many patients, particularly urban citizens, know that AIDS and cancer, among others, are diseases that are difficult to treat with biomedicine in a resource-poor environment. The only alternatives they have at their disposal, then, are "modern" healing marabouts. These healers at the forefront of modern life are poised to take advantage of this opportunity. On private radio, they make use of numerous advertising spots and time slots ranging from 15 minutes to an hour, during which they display all their healing knowledge.

These modern healers also have mobile phones and business cards at their disposal to insure them against the anonymity of their forebears. Some have come from the interior of the country to better promote their services through the media and in the capital, but the vast majority are from Niamey and its surroundings. Practitioners in Nigeria have contributed greatly to the advent of this innovation in communication. They were the first to take to the airways to reach the public. All use the honorific "Doctor" (e.g., Dr. Abiola, Dr. Mashood, Dr. Bouhary, Dr. Sanoussi, Dr. Oumar) and feature interviews with patients they have cured of illnesses ranging from the minor to the seemingly incurable. In addition, the print media grants them more and more space for advertising, interviews, and testimonials.

Maraboutic treatments are based on the combined or separate use of holy water, amulets, and short blessings said to show results overnight. Often the marabout recites incantations derived from Qur'anic writings or *hadiths* for long hours in the woman's presence. He also blows on her intermittently. Other components of their remedies include honey, sheep's liver, and the powders of certain plants. Holy water, called *hantum hari* (Z) and *ruwan allo* or *rubutu* (H), is obtained when the Qur'anic text a marabout writes on a wooden tablet (*allo* [H]) or on paper is washed off and the water is collected in a container to drink. A woman seeking motherhood may be instructed to consume this holy water over several weeks or even months. Some marabouts prescribe a mixture composed of sheep's liver and holy water. The woman has two choices for obtaining the organ. She either goes to a butcher she trusts, or she sacrifices the animal herself to be sure she has the liver, which she must then bring back to the marabout. She will cook the liver in the same holy water mentioned above. Once cooked, she must eat it all. This treatment is considered to be effective after one to three trials.

This same holy water can also be used for curative baths. The patient washes herself with *hantum hari*, which she has carefully poured into a gourd that has never been used. Sometimes she must also recite a few suras and other holy formulae taught to her by the marabout beforehand. Specific postures are also dictated during this ritual cleansing, such as sitting, squatting, or standing. Women who hope to become mothers also wear amulets on certain parts of the body, particularly the waist or the arm or in the hair.

Following the instructions from the marabout she consults (e.g., incantations to recite, postures to hold), a woman seeking to become pregnant performs prayer vigils periodically or over a certain duration (three, seven, or nine days, for example) to exorcise the evil in her. Fasting is prescribed as part of the treatment for infertility in conjunction with night prayers. As with the lengths of prayer vigils, odd numbers are favored—fasts must occur over three or seven days.

Traditional Healers

The esoteric nature of the practices of traditional healers presents a major challenge when collecting data, but most healers' remedies are derived from herbal medicine. Most often, traditional healers use the placenta of a ruminant animal such as a sheep, goat, or heifer that has just given birth and add the placenta to various mixtures made generally of plants. Then, depending on the case, it is either consumed by the patient or rubbed against her stomach. Similarly, rituals to free an infertile woman from her enchantment are carried out on the banks of the Niger River, where various offerings are made to water spirits. Some are said to be costly in both time and emotional resources. But is not one willing to endure any hardship when one wants children? Some women agree to defy the prescriptions of their religion (for example, Islam, which is strongly opposed to animist ceremonies) to overcome infertility. Such rituals may require baths, denudation, and rites of spirit possession called *bori*.

Typically, women indigenous to the region are directed to perform rituals rooted in the local landscape. Alone or in the presence of the prescribing healer and third parties, an infertile woman is told to wash herself at the base of a termite mound with a mixture whose chemical composition remains difficult to pinpoint. Termite mounds are said to be reservoirs that collect the curses and negative attributes present in a person. This therapeutic bath allows infertile women suspected of having committed or having been the target of malicious acts to get rid of the evil. One of my respondents, still hoping for a child, recounts a time when she had a bathing ceremony:

> We went far from Niamey in the middle of the night with the *zimma* [a Zarma healer] and two of his [female] disciples. We went to the bottom of a termite mound I'd identified myself two days earlier with one of my friends and my brother, who was driving the car. There, I got completely undressed and sat next to the termite mound, facing away from it. The *zimma* sprinkled me with a foul-smelling liquid while reciting incantations I didn't understand. It looked like it had blood in it. The two disciples took turns walking around the termite mound and rubbing my face with white powder. (Madame IM, 43 years old, childless, Balafon district)

Subfertile women may also seek treatment for infertility through a spirit possession cult.[2] Such cults offer a sense of community, protection, and possibility to women who otherwise experience their infertility as the cause of their marginalization. If they are initiated, they may take part in possession dances that are expressly organized for them to learn to accommodate a spirit and to persuade it to unblock the conception of a child. The spirit may then require specific gifts and sacrifices. Like maraboutic and traditional therapies, possession treatments are often accompanied by the sacrifice of chickens, small ruminants (e.g., ewes, goats, or sheep), and sometimes even large ruminants.

Informants who had sought remedies for their infertility in coastal countries including Benin, Togo, or Ghana spoke of being stripped of clothing. Perhaps this call for nudity is linked to a notion of an original state without sin, without defilement; and stripping the infertile woman naked is understood to return her to this state. Denudation can be partial or total. Sometimes there was a simulation of the sexual act, perhaps staging future sexual encounters that are fruitful. Or perhaps this simulated sexual act marks a break away from all prior attempts, which were in vain. It is not impossible that such rituals are also practiced in Niger, particularly among populations that have not converted to Islam.

2. Editor's note: Research on such cults is abundant (Rasmussen 2012; Stoller 1995; Masquelier 2001; Pasian 2010; Monfouga-Nicolas 1972; Echard 1989).

When infertility treatments fail to yield positive results, how do men and women manage their condition? What practical arrangements and palliative measures are used? What are the socio-psychological implications of different interventions? Michel Adam notes that "although sterility is an individual drama, it is shared customs and traditions that are largely responsible for resolving the problem of childless marriages" (1994: 5). How this social undertaking plays out depends on the context and is often subject to change. In general, family-level solutions and alternatives are those that are socially acceptable.

In light of the data I collected, there are four modes of managing infertility. In order of significance and frequency they are polygamy, fostering or *confiage*,[3] divorce, and adultery. These are not mutually exclusive strategies for managing infertility. A woman's inability to conceive may be concealed by the presence of children of one or more co-wives. A woman may in certain cases benefit from "substitute children" by welcoming the children of kin or of classificatory kinship. In the most extreme cases, which are seldom reported and assiduously hidden, a lover might produce children (without the social father's knowledge or with his relatives' complicity) for a woman who does not have any of her own.

Polygamy

The couple that is childless by choice, a family model sometimes seen in developed countries, is virtually unknown in Sahelian Muslim and Nigerien societies where—despite the social, economic, and political changes underway—women are and remain "always mothers-before-all" (Lacoste-Dujardin [1985] 1996: 67). When motherhood does not occur in the anticipated time frame, society turns to polygamy as a means of managing infertility. This type of response is considered an adaptive way to ease a woman's frustration with her lack of biological children. The integration of a woman via polygamy can take place in two main forms, which I refer to as "anterior integration" and "posterior integration." In the first model, the

3. Editor's note: The French term *confiage* comes from the verb *confier*, which can be translated as "to entrust [something/someone] to [someone]." Here, we translate it as "fostering," a practice that is to be distinguished from adoption, which, as HM explains, is not an option for Muslims in the local understanding of Islamic religious practice.

infertile woman is the first wife. Her husband takes a second wife after she is presumed sterile. In the second model, the woman who has not conceived in her first marriage marries an already-married man; in this case she is the second, third, or fourth wife. The posterior integration of an infertile woman into a polygamous household or into a household already full of children constitutes marital security and even, in some respects, proof of social rehabilitation. The infertile woman's new husband recognizes her as such and marries her despite this disadvantage. The husband has already had the opportunity to prove his "paternity" with his other wife or wives.[4] He thus knows that he is assured descendants.

The system of polygamy—in contrast with divorce—provides a woman marital protection. When in a polygamous marriage, a woman's sterility can be clearly established in some cases; and in other cases, a woman's presumed sterility can be disproven. According to some of the women I interviewed, "the practice of polygamy is considered beneficial to the wife" for two main reasons. For one, polygamy can relieve her of responsibility for the couple's infertility; if her co-wife does not give birth within an acceptable time frame, responsibility will be passed on to the husband. Additionally, the arrival of the new wife can help the first (ostensibly sterile) wife to conceive. It is said that the first wife's desire to have a child might be reignited simply through jealousy.

A woman presumed sterile could therefore become pregnant "out of jealousy," after having witnessed her co-wife's pregnancy:

> In a home with no births, the man is asked to enter a second marriage. It's the best way for them to find out which of them is "deficient." With a little luck, her husband's remarriage will be a good opportunity for the first wife, as she might still become pregnant. Or it's when the second wife gets pregnant that the other will also become pregnant through jealousy. In that way, the two women will become pregnant at the same time. . . . Personally, I have a sister who experienced something similar. After her first child, she went twenty years without conceiving. In order for my sister to become pregnant again, her husband had to remarry and her co-wife to become pregnant a month after the marriage. . . . This is why we say, "the stomach is jealous" (*gunde ga canse* [Z]). Without jealousy, how do you explain how a woman who's been childless for twenty years ends up conceiving. . . . It's in these cases that the Zarma say "*gunde ga canse*." (Madame

---

4. Polygamy is no longer recognized in some countries, particularly Tunisia (Tichit 2009: 9). This can weaken the standing of the infertile woman as she might simply be repudiated rather than being joined by one or more co-wives.

GH, 55 years old, four children, companion of a woman giving birth, Gaweye district)

Whatever the integration model, it is meant to promote a distribution of parental roles between fertile and infertile wives within the same marital unit. However, on closer inspection, this dynamic is not always effective due to the almost permanently prevailing climate of strong or latent conflict in polygamous households. As rivalry is, according to Sylvie Fainzang, "a structural feature of the polygamous institution" (1991: 98), many childless women say they are goaded and often persecuted by their co-wife-mothers.

It sometimes happens that my co-wife prevents her children from going to do my shopping and she indirectly makes comments like "a mother for each child and a child for each mother." (Madame IM, 43 years old, childless, Balafon district)

Despite the rivalry between co-wives, many infertile women lead "normal lives" wherein threats of divorce and repudiation are less present than in cases of monogamy. As Yannick Jaffré writes, a co-wife "can also become a 'palliative,' offering the group a child and preventing the infertile woman from being repudiated or from fleeing to return to her family rather than remain in an untenable situation" (1997: 13). Infertile women may accept conflict with their co-wives in the hope of enjoying more favor in their relationship with the husband.

For some infertile women, polygamy ensures marital security more than it grants them parental rights over the children of their co-wives. A fertile wife's main weapon of self-validation is her children. Differential treatment between wives is commonplace in polygamous households. As a result, the infertile woman is often excluded from the family structure. The husband prefers giving gifts to fertile wives. Even with reproductive parity, co-wives rarely benefit from the same treatment (e.g., emotional, material, statutory) from their husband.

From this perspective, polygamy is for many infertile women an alternative status to being unmarried, which remains highly stigmatized. A woman must always remain under a male guardian: first familial, then marital (Héritier 1996). An independent woman, whether divorced, widowed, or never married, is assumed to be "loose."[5] As a result, many infertile women

5. This category of women is generally designated in Zarma by the pejorative expression *wey-kuuru*. Olivier de Sardan (1984) provides more detail on the term: *wey* means woman, and *kuuru* indicates vacant, available. This term also evokes prostitution.

resign themselves to the arrival of one or more co-wives under the marital roof or to leaving their marriages to take refuge in a polygamous home.

In Cameroon, Tichit observed that polygamy is one of the main strategies used to compensate for the absence of children in a marriage. Polygamy sometimes comes about as a result of the family's involvement:

> Family control does not simply intervene in the choice of the spouse but also in the monitoring of her fertility. Once married, any fertile dysfunction causes conjugal difficulties and arouses the concern of the family circle. At best, this results in the arrival of a co-wife selected by the husband's family. . . . A simple delay in the constitution of offspring, or the accumulation of miscarriages or infantile death compromises the young woman's status, no matter the legitimacy of her marital status. A fertility considered insufficient condemns a woman to polygamy, or worse . . . to singledom [as a result of being repudiated]. (2009: 8–9)

This family interference can sometimes be fairly dramatic: some men find themselves presented with "ready-to-wed" wives without having pursued any aspect of the remarriage themselves. These young brides who are "imposed" on men generally come from their extended family, whereas the first wives, now presumed sterile, were chosen from outside. When a man is reluctant to take another wife because his first wife has no children, his family tries to confront him with a fait accompli, as in the case of someone I will refer to as ZIM.

ZIM, who left on leave for a few (four) days, brought back with his luggage an unusual package: a new wife. His first wife, after two and a half years of marriage, had not yet had children. Annoyed by this situation, his parents (living in the village) had arranged a marriage with the daughter of ZIM's father's best friend. Unbeknown to him, his parents had taken care of all the formalities surrounding the marriage. Then, under the pretext of an extremely serious problem, his parents asked him to return to the village as a matter of urgency; the rest is clear. This type of family interference leaves the underlying issue of infertility unresolved.

Fostering or *Confiage*

Hadjia SM was 48 years old in November 2006. Married to her cousin for 29 years, she had never had a child. Her husband took two other wives. The first gave birth to six children, while the second is the mother of four. At the age of 32, with her husband's agreement, Hadjia was entrusted with the care of one of her nieces and her youngest brother. She also raised one of her first co-wife's daughters, as well as one of her sisters-in-law. Her first two "gifted" children are now married. It was only after several unsuccessful treatment attempts that she decided to raise children from the "family." Hadjia SM still plans to take in one or two more of her close relatives' children.

I use the terms "fostering," "gift," "placement," and "*confiage*" interchangeably to designate the same general practice, even if the specific provisions in particular instances may differ. For reasons I will discuss, the term "adoption" is not applicable here.

Certain forms of sterility management, because they are more or less in line with dominant social values, allow for a re-establishment of the social order initially disturbed by the "lack of children." Laurence Pourchez notes that among Creole women in Réunion, the transfer of children may take place "between women who have children and women who do not; they forego abortion and the unwanted child is entrusted to a woman with few children or to a sterile woman. This compensatory practice is thus close to the role given to 'fostering' in African societies where, in certain cases, children are given with priority to infertile women" (2002: 92). Pourchez argues that in the Creole context infertile women may thereby regain social recognition as mothers. This kind of re-establishment of balance is mentioned by Suzanne Lallemand as well, who notes that children circulate frequently in Africa (1988a: 135). She distinguishes between exclusive adoptions (in which the rights of the biological parents are replaced by those of the adoptive parents) and inclusive adoptions (in which the rights of the biological parents coexist with those of the adoptive parents) (Lallemand 1988b). This first, "full" adoption is more common in Western sociocultural contexts, and the second, "simple" adoption, is more typical in Africa. Bonnet, whose research falls within a sociocultural context similar to that studied by Lallemand, observes that this transfer of children takes place "to the benefit of women who are no longer in the reproductive cycle and to the detriment of those who, on the contrary, ensure the fertility of the lineage" (Bonnet 1988: 104).

In Niger the sterility or underfertility of some women prompts the circulation of children in the form of *confiage* or giving a child to be fostered by families or individuals lacking their own descendants. In a way, fostering is the African counterpart of adoption in the West. Full adoption in its strict sense is uncommon in Niger, in large part due to Islamic social values. The practice of full adoption with rights of inheritance is not endorsed by the Muslim religion. In Sura 33 of the Qur'an (*Al-ahzab*, The Clans, The Coalition, The Combined Forces), in verse 4, it is stated "He has not made your adopted children your own children."

Those who provide children—generally relatives—provide both men and women with the offspring necessary for their mental and psychosocial well-being, often at the cost of marital conflict:

> My wife was opposed to the idea of giving one of our children to my older sister who never had one. We had difficult times for several weeks. (OS, 37 years old, six children, welder, Lazaret district)

In addition, according to popular belief, taking in or spending time with the children of others (a family member, a friend, or, as mentioned above, even a co-wife) might trigger a woman's maternal desire to positive effect. An infertile woman is often referred to as a woman whose "sleeping maternal cells" finally wake up in order to conceive:

> Just being in contact with children can increase a woman's chances for pregnancy. Before, our ancestors always advised a woman who was slow to conceive to welcome children into her home. (Madame GH, 55 years old, four children, companion of a woman giving birth, Gaweye district)

It seems that for a woman considered infertile, her mothering capacities are developed through taking in a child, as her desire to have a child becomes more acute (Stork 1999). This circulation of children among friends and family highlights the forms of familial solidarity that emerge in interdependent relationships and goes beyond the individualistic framework of infertility care.

Yet this compensation through the placement of children never erases and never obscures the infertile woman's biological "disadvantage." One is always a "fictive," "partial," or "quasi" parent, to use the terminology set by Josiane Massard in her study of the circulation of children in Malaysia (1988).[6] In Niger, the local terms that designate "fostered" children illustrate the temporary nature of this compensation fairly well. In Hausa, the entrusted child is called *dan riko*, *dan* = son [of] and *riko* = custody; the expression therefore literally means "the child of custody" or "the borrowed child" and, in Zarma, *ta ka biiri* (literally, "keep and raise" or "take and raise"). *Biiri* means "to raise, to educate" (Bernard and White-Kaba 1994: 33).

What's more, the incessant question "Do you have children?" that no man or woman can escape cannot be answered (as it might be in the West) without distinguishing between fostered and biological children. This

6. Massard borrows these terms from Goody (1969).

question refers exclusively to the biological children to whom one has given birth. The biological child is designated by the expressions *ize-gunde* (literally, "stomach-son" [Z]) and *dan ciki* ("son of the belly" [H]):

> A *dan riko* ultimately remains his parents' child. He cannot be otherwise. Whenever the need arises, he'll prove this and return home. (Madame MY, 52 years old, mother of nine children, Gaweye district)

The children of others, no matter how obtained, remain the children of their biological parents and only temporarily those of their foster parents. While a person to whom a child is entrusted enjoys a delegation of parental rights or custody, biological ties continue to predominate. The foster parent assumes only social parenting roles. Fostering never erases one's biological inability to give birth. In the context of his study of stigma, Erving Goffman notes that "Where [correction of a perceived defect] is possible, what often results is not the acquisition of fully normal status, but a transformation of self from someone with a particular blemish into someone with a record of having corrected a particular blemish."[7] The stigmatized may be reminded of the stigma through "taunts, teasing, ostracism, and fights" (Goffman 1963: 33). This is true for one woman whose sisters-in-law kept reminding her that she was "surrounded by the children of others":

> Everyone knows that the two children who live under my roof are from my family: one is my nephew and the other is my little sister. Despite their presence in the house, people continue to wonder when I'll finally have "my own child" (*dana na kai na* [H]). The children of others protect you around those who don't know you. But for everyone else who's been around you every day for a long time, your inability to give birth is the first and only thing that jumps out at them. My sisters-in-law often remind me of this indirectly. (Madame HS2, 31 years old, childless, Yantala district)

In this interview, we can see that *dana na kai na* ("my own child," or *ay bon ize* [Z], literally, "a child of one's own blood") is more desirable, more valued than *dan riko* or *ta ka biiri*. The reception of "temporary children" does not definitively liberate the childless woman, who continues to feel a sense of deficiency. The fostering of children, while allowing infertile women to assume a long-awaited maternal parental function, does not

---

7. Editor's note: Wherever HM quoted from a French translation of a text written originally in English we have sought out the original language and cited the English publication. Goffman (1963: 9).

enable them to gain the status of a "complete woman" who has given birth. Simone de Beauvoir's famous phrase in *The Second Sex*, "one is not born, but rather becomes, a woman" is shown in all its meaning here (1973: 301). The construction of femininity is a process that remains unfinished, even unstarted, for some of the women who experience primary sterility. "Acting as if one is a mother" therefore does not have the same meaning as "truly being a mother."

In short, in Niamey, as elsewhere in Niger, infertile women welcome "substitute children" into their homes despite not being able to access the status of full mothers fully and unambiguously. A reflection made to me by a medical intern during an informal interview summarizes quite clearly the distinction that is drawn between a biological mother (who is also the social mother in most cases) and a social mother who has not experienced the physiological, anatomical, and psychological changes of pregnancy:

> You know, ma'am, many people think real mothers draw their children from of their own wombs while foster mothers gain . . . excuse the expression . . . gain "ready-made children" [*enfants clés-en-mains*] thanks to the pity and charity of the former. (Medical intern, Central Maternity Hospital)[8]

For Thérèse Locoh the *confiage* of children is akin to a practice of "load sharing": "a mother who has many children can 'shed' some by giving them to another family for a more or less long duration. Conversely, a 'sub-fertile' woman will 'borrow' children from her sisters, aunts, and cousins to keep her company. There is frequently a circulation of children to allow a better distribution of the load they represent" (1984: 145).

Many fostering arrangements in urban areas are performed according to quite selective criteria, often economic. Madame HS4, married to a polygamous man, had never been able to "fully adopt" a child:

> I've taken in children from my family twice. But neither of them stayed more than two years. They were called back home after a while. I'm sure they wouldn't have done this if I was wealthy. One of my cousins has been entrusted with children for life without even needing to ask. She already has her own children and three others who were given to her just like that, while I still have a hard time

---

8. Editor's note: The French expression *clés-en-mains* originally referred to purchasing a finished house rather than having it built to specifications, a usage that is suggestive of something accomplished with less effort. A close business English equivalent today would be "turnkey" or "end-to-end." A more colloquial translation might be "pre-fab."

getting any. She's rich and works for a company; that's not my case. If I'd had brothers or sisters, things might've been different. You come out of the same womb as them, they sympathize more with your pain, and they're always ready to help you. (Madame HS4, 41 years old, childless, Zabarkan district)

Madame HH expresses herself in roughly the same terms:

If you're rich, your children's playground is invaded without your asking. Otherwise, you often have to beg people to entrust one of their children to you, and other times, you have to humble yourself. (Madame HH, 37 years old, childless, Collège Mariama district)

In some cases, for as long as they hope to have children, couples reject family or external interference. Few resort to fostering as a solution to infertility during the first months or years of their marriage.

I've been married for three years. I still believe in my chances of having a child. I'm still young and I have a lot of hope. Another person's child can often cause problems. Things have changed; parents can tear themselves apart because of their children. In any case, for now I continue to wait, I'm not in a hurry, and we'll see what happens. (Madame FC, 26 years old, childless, Lamordé district)

On the one hand, for some women, it is after several of their own unsuccessful attempts to become pregnant that they call on the children of others. The idea of fostering only becomes an option for them when they have mourned their inability to become biological mothers. On the other hand, some family members who provide children follow an equally rational logic and do not wait for the need for a child to become apparent within the family or one of its members before offering their "charitable" services to "those without child." Santiago-Delefosse (1995) remarks that other women refuse to consider taking in children because for them it means both taking on a debt (assuming a duty) and acknowledging their lack of offspring.

Some infertile women like Hadjia SM, cited above, made fostering their life's work. Similarly, Baba of Karo, a Hausa-speaking woman whose life story was recorded by Mary Smith (1954) in the 1950s, fostered the children of many different family members including children of co-wives. Baba was married at least four times in her search for a fertile marriage. Her repeated marriages illustrate the historical depth of the instability and precariousness of life for childless women in this region.

Divorce and Remarriage

Numerous studies show the predominance of marital instability in infertile households (Thiriat 1998; Erny 1988; Locoh 1984). The separation of spouses as a result of infertility is common in Nigerien society. Among Yoruba couples in Nigeria, where some of the values are similar to those in Niger, Winny Koster indicates that a legitimate cause for divorce—for men and women alike—is infertility (2003: 92). In their introduction to an edited collection on infertility in Africa, Ties Boerma and Zaida Mgalla observed that "women who do not bear children are often divorced, have multiple life-time partners, and are therefore apt to have sexual intercourse with fertile partners at some point in their lives" (2001: 15–16). Individuals, in particular women, who struggle to conceive are likely to experience marital instability and a relatively high number of different marriages (Héritier 1984: 137). Divorce seems to occur in cases of impatience manifested by one or both spouses, especially if the idea of polygamy is not entertained.

> I'm on my second marriage, but I'm sure I'll be on my third soon. My husband has no regard for me. I continue to live under his roof in the hope that one day I'll have a child, or if not, be protected by marriage . . . so people from outside have to respect you, so they don't think you're a free woman. You know how people think here. But the longer I stay, the worse it gets. Usually, he hardly even looks at me. It's rare that he touches me; only when things aren't going well with the other [co-wife]. (Madame HS2, 31 years old, childless, Yantala district)

Infertility can lead to marital nomadism, which sometimes does not end until old age, almost on the eve of menopause.

Adultery

Adultery has often been mentioned as a way of testing the fertility of both women and men. The secretive character of adultery in general, and particularly the social dismissal of male adultery, nevertheless makes any investigation on the subject difficult. Multiple partners for married and unmarried men are tolerated, if not encouraged. The extra-marital adventures of a man who has not had children in his current marriage favor his eventual marriage to the mistress he impregnates. Women testing their reproductive skills are faced with two scenarios: either they finally conceive and stop feeling guilty and at the same time cover their husband's assumed sterility, or these attempts remain unsuccessful and they become convinced of their condition. It is nearly impossible to collect first-hand accounts directly from men and women who have such stories. I was, however, told in great detail about the marital adventures of "others." It was sometimes possible for me to deduce the parties involved through triangulation.

Case Study: Madame Malam H, the "Adulterous" Mother

I met Madame Malam H, known as "S," in recovery at the Talladjé Maternity Ward where she had just given birth. She was married to a childless polygamist. She offered up her opinion on infertility, as well as the socially condemned strategies that some people employ to ensure themselves children:

> Infertility is a hard thing for a woman to bear. She's often forced unwillingly to either take the blame for her husband's infertility or to find other socially prohibited solutions. Because many sterile men escape social stigma by knowing how to exploit unsuspected ruses, some women without children choose not to sit idly by. They'd go to the devil if it meant getting pregnant (*i ga ba ibilisi gana ga te gunde* [Z]). So they're willing to try condemned practices. I knew two women, initially considered sterile, who ended up having children. Other men are the biological fathers. They cheated on their husbands because they were never able to have children with other women (wives or mistresses). Their husbands turn a blind eye because it benefits them.

Madame Malam H's husband never had a child with his two other wives, wives who he quickly divorced when Madam Malam H became pregnant. The mistress he had kept for three years to test his procreative capacities had also not conceived. I met acquaintances of the couple who confirmed the main elements of this story (a sister-in-law of Madam Malam H, a half-sister of the husband, someone from the neighborhood, and one of the former co-wives of Madame Malam H). One of Madame Malam H's co-wives said the following to me:

> I stayed with Malam H for three years without a child. He married S at the end of our third year of marriage. After 14 months, nothing had happened. He took a third wife, still childless. And it was in this situation that one good morning we miraculously found out that S was pregnant. In that moment, I personally understood that I wasn't sterile, and that something strange was happening in the house. S had never been a well-behaved quiet woman. Seriously, she never had been. Before her marriage to Malam H, S had apparently had several abortions.

I learned this through mutual acquaintances. Faced with this knowledge, I made the decision to divorce my husband before he had the same idea. He agreed [to the divorce] without hesitation, and in the same stroke he asked his newest wife to leave as well. I remarried only two months after the period of *viduité*.[9] I had a child the same year, and I'm currently pregnant. My other co-wife hasn't remarried, but she gave birth last year. Do you understand? Malam H is sterile; he has to admit it. If he refuses, he'll answer to God.

Some men can save face through the adultery of their wives. Although socially and religiously proscribed, adultery in the case of infertility serves practical ends. As Héritier notes, "from the very fact that a man can always be credited with descendants who come to him from his legitimate wives, male sterility does not in itself matter, and therefore it is not at all necessary to identify or recognize it as such" (1996: 78). Danièle Kintz also refers to "utilitarian" adultery among Fulanis: "When a woman has no children, before concluding that she is sterile, she tries other partners, whether within the context of remarriage or that of adultery. This approach can even be organized by the couple in mutual agreement, with a friend of the husband providing his sexual services. This is the Fulani technique of natural insemination" (1987: 139). Along similar lines Koster (2003: 282) comments that in the Yoruba context in Nigeria a woman who wishes to remain by her husband's side could try to become pregnant with a different man, but she must do so in secret for the child to be accepted by her husband and his kin.

Notwithstanding the ultra-clandestine nature of adultery, the quiet complicity of others covers the participants. Very often, people around the culpable woman will suspect the illegitimacy of her conception. The family is faced with a quasi-dilemma: to reveal or to keep silent about what is normally called deviant behavior. Keeping quiet seems the better option for the man and his relatives if, despite numerous sexual attempts, he has not succeeded in impregnating a woman. Revealing a married woman's adultery can be a source of humiliation for the man and his relatives. This is because such a situation challenges the ideal of the virile man.

9. Editor's note: This period, referred to in French as *le délai de viduité*, refers to a legally imposed period that divorced or widowed women are expected to observe before contracting a subsequent marriage in order to avoid ambiguity in paternity rights and obligations. French civil law required a nine-month delay until advances in paternity testing prompted its abrogation in 2004 (law 2004-439 of May 26, 2004). Such laws are still relevant in much of the Muslim world, the "count" of the delay ('idda) being typically three menstrual periods.

Among other factors supposed to prove a married woman's infidelity, people I interviewed cited the color of an infant's skin and certain facial features upon which much speculation is made in the first weeks following the child's birth. Some parents and friends seek to console themselves over the extra-marital origins of the pregnancy through the child's resemblance to a member of either family such as brothers, sisters, uncles, aunts, and grandparents. This explains how the adultery, when committed with someone within the inner circle of the women's in-laws, unless they are discovered, generally passes unsuspected. This interview excerpt illustrates a case of this phenomenon:

One of my former neighbors, a mother of three beautiful boys, made them all with her husband Elhadji's uncle. Her husband is infertile, even if he doesn't dare admit it. The resemblance between Elhadji, his uncle, and these children is striking. Elhadji's a very rich man. And the rich, you know, aren't satisfied with just one woman. He subsequently took two other wives who were much younger than the first. But none of them gave birth. Not even a miscarriage. One, who suspected her husband was sterile from the start, divorced him after eighteen months. Now she's the mother of two children with her new husband. As for my former neighbor Elhadji, he's consoled himself with this explanation: that he suffers from secondary infertility. After allegedly undergoing tests in Côte d'Ivoire, he was told that he'd become sterile not long ago. . . . *Astakfirullah!* [May God forgive me]. This couple lived next to us for twelve years. And I noticed the complicity between the lady and her handsome uncle. He lived in a village near Niamey. He used any pretext to come to his nephew's house, including watching over the house during Elhadji's long and interminable business trips. The notorious uncle's wife often had fits of jealousy because of her husband's attitude toward his beautiful niece. Now she's just turned thirty-seven but no longer gives birth. And you know what? Her lover has died! It was only after his uncle's death that Elhadji revealed his secondary sterility. It's not a coincidence! Lots of people have talked about this in secret. For a while, this story was the talk of the neighborhood. (Hadjia A, 52 years old, Banifandou district)

Marriage between cousins (parallel or crossed) is a common practice in Niger. In these cases, whether the woman has sexual relations with her own close relatives or those of her husband, her child will resemble the rest of the family. The adage "he who says nothing agrees" is apt in the appreciation of this compromise. This type of tacit accommodation is not quite the same as the system of "loaning" the wife to a friend or the practice of "circumstantial" levirate marriage that Odile Journet (1991) noted among the Joola people of Casamance.

Women are not passive in the face of men's refusal to acknowledge their sterility. Sometimes women in-laws conspire to overcome the sterility of a man, as Mgalla and Boerma (2002: 198) suggest occurs in Tanzania. In this regard, adultery, far from being a purely individual initiative for the management of infertility, can be socially organized to compensate for the couple's absence of children. A maxim common in Niger tacitly tolerates the adultery committed by a woman who becomes pregnant: "a thief has no children." Here, the thief is the lover of the adulterous woman. Though conceived in an extra-marital setting, the child belongs to the legally married couple. This is an advantage that social and Islamic jurisprudence have accorded to married men.

CONCLUSION

The different methods of managing infertility are sometimes closely intertwined. Women having multiple partnerships (following successive divorces or because of adultery) may be linked to the popular theory of blood incompatibility. The conviction that her blood and that of her husband cannot fuse together can lead a woman to undergo successive marriages, in the hope of constituting a "matched couple." The same logic can push her, while staying with the same husband, to break the rules of marital fidelity on one or more occasions. In addition, the practices of polygamy and fostering can go together. An infertile woman can take in the children of others while living in a polygamous household.

Polygamy in a Muslim marriage, however, does not guarantee a childless woman marital security. To "secure herself," the Arab woman must, Bouhdiba observes, play the cards "of pregnancy, breastfeeding, and education" wisely for her own well-being (2001: 278). In such contexts, as in Niger, children are mediating factors, not only between the husband and wife but also between the couple and the husband's family. The ostracism of infertile women, often combined with social marginality, can be a source of great suffering.

In my research among practitioners and patients about the different modes of infertility management within familial, popular, and medical environments, success stories were rare. Sometimes one recalled distant echoes of a feat attributed to this or that specialist, constituting their sole basis for publicity. Some individuals yearning for a child of their own have alternated between traditional, popular, and biomedical methods. Others have combined them or used them simultaneously. Some women have been able to conceive at the end of these hybrid and syncretic journeys, but the real causes of these successes are unknown. The marabout or the healer is primarily credited with the success. The medical system, except when it is the only site where a woman seeks treatment, is almost never attributed with the resolution of the unfortunate situation. In Chapter 5, it will become clearer why this is the case.

CHAPTER 3

Varieties of Infertility

This chapter presents a social typology of infertility by drawing upon my conversations with six women with varied but illustrative experiences. I will present the life stories of women who are sterile, women who have given birth to children who died at a young age, and women who are subfertile (or hypofertile). In Nigeria, Winny Koster (2003) notes, the "Yoruba . . . differentiate between types of infertility: never having conceived, never having delivered a live birth, not having living children, and having only one or two children" (p. 262). The experiences of women who have never had children, who have had children who did not survive, and who have had few children should not be conflated. Given the diversity of their circumstances, childless women may be better described as "women with various fertility conditions."

These individual journeys are suggestive of the common struggles of women seeking a sense of identity and self-worth. Their experiences illustrate an essential theme in this book: that the social attainment of womanhood in Niger occurs through motherhood. In local constructions, womanhood and motherhood are intertwined such that one takes on its meaning in relation to the other. Examining portraits of women with a variety of fertility conditions enables me to bring together a range of experiences that nevertheless overlap. The experiences are distinct, but they are not isolated. These narratives reveal the twists and turns, the good and the bad, that characterize the sexual and reproductive trajectories of women facing fertility constraints. They also uncover the battles women wage to improve their social status as "childless women."

Yearning and Refusal. Hadiza Moussa, Edited by Alice J. Kang and Barbara M. Cooper, Oxford University Press.
© Oxford University Press 2023. DOI: 10.1093/oso/9780197662113.003.0004

STERILITY: AN "EMPTY" LIFE LACKING CONTINUITY

Case Study 1: Fanta, 38 Years Old, Never Conceived, "a Stranger in My Own Home"

Fanta has beautiful features that make her unforgettable. She said she was 38 years old at the time of our first meeting, but if she hadn't said otherwise, one would think her barely in her thirties. Her first marriage took place when she was 15 and a half, and she had just started high school in Zinder a few months before. Her husband, who she had "never loved nor chosen," already had one wife who was a mother of five. According to Fanta, her husband unilaterally divorced her after a turbulent and depressing 27 months of marriage for not having conceived a child.

Sobbing, Fanta recounts these last words from her first husband, who constantly denigrated her in the presence of others:

> You're not a woman. I feed and clothe you for no reason, because you aren't even capable of continuing my name. You're a waste of my time and money. Disappear from my life and take your bad luck with you. Your stomach only knows how to gobble up food. I didn't marry you for pleasure; I already have one wife for that and there are plenty more out there. If you only knew how to do something with your two hands. You sleep and you eat, and your whole life is limited to these two activities. Nothing more! Go!

Humiliating his wife had become a habit, especially in front of his family. The year after her divorce, Fanta enrolled in secondary school, received her BEPC, and entered the École Normale in Tahoua.[1] She graduated two years later as a primary school teacher, which she considers as having "won one round of the fight" because she is able to meet her "daily needs without anyone's help." Four years later she remarried, this time to a divorced man with one child. Her life is no better because after one year living together, she finds herself with a co-wife younger than herself, who quickly became pregnant and attracted most of her husband's attention. Hardship after hardship followed, she says, of a "rather cynical, but also quite underhanded" nature. This is how she describes her situation:

> I began to feel like a stranger in my own home. I moved and did things with much less confidence than before. Yes, I was no longer sure of myself. I felt

---

1. Editor's note: The Brevet d'Études du Premier Cycle is roughly equivalent to a high school diploma. The École Normal in Tahoua is a state-funded teacher training school.

diminished, incomplete. . . . One way or another, my husband reminds me that I'm less important than anyone else in the house, including his relatives or the children of his friends who are our guests. My husband treats me and my co-wife very differently (*kullum yana bambanci tsakaninmu, ni da kishiyata* [H]), which makes my position more unbearable. All the little gifts that my husband brings to the house are given in priority to my co-wife, to his child, and to his niece who has come to live with us. I feel like I'm no longer treated like a person. It's a question of pride—I have to leave him. I've lost all my self-esteem. I only ever receive sudden and fleeting attention from my husband when we have guests, especially when they're my family. He hasn't fully rejected me, because he wants me to tire and discourage myself and leave our shared home on my own.

At the time of our engagement, I'd told him I had problems conceiving, and at the time he was so blinded by his love for me that he'd sworn faithfulness, promised me the moon. He promised to do all he could, including artificial insemination so I could have a child in my life. It's not even available in Niamey, but he promised it. After the wedding, he only went to the gynecologist with me once, and funded treatments for just one year. Then he told me to take care of myself, saying, "You have to take your fate into your own hands. I did what I could. I can't do more. I have other priorities." Meanwhile, my co-wife gave birth again. She had twins.

Ever since, my husband swears only by her, sees only her, listens only to her. He often calls her "*lantarki*" to provoke or to humiliate me.[2] She represents the fortune I never had. In short, my husband doesn't have the slightest regard for me. This ordeal has been going on for a little over 10 years. I know I'll eventually leave him. All my measly teaching salary goes toward examinations and fertility treatments but without success. They've given me many traditional and maraboutic remedies. Marabouts have told me to fast for days, and I have. Multiple times I have fasted for seven days and at the end made a sacrifice of chickens, sheep, beignets, sugar, fresh milk, etc. Often, I have stayed awake during the night, reciting various verses from the Qur'an that the marabout had given to me beforehand. A friend suggested that I go see a great *bori* leader. He gave me multiple potions made of powders and herbs. Then he asked me to take a nighttime bath at the foot of a termite mound. I performed this ritual three nights in a row. I've also participated in *bori* dances of possession to exorcise the evil that inhabits me and keeps me from conceiving. In addition, I've drunk almost nothing but *ruwan allo* ("holy water" [H]). I go to the marabout twice a week for it. . . . And all these things, I've paid for with my own money. My

2. Editor's note: In Hausa *lantarki* refers to a microwave oven. Her co-wife is a newer model who "cooks quickly."

parents are poor, they can only pray for me. Aside from that, I have no support. I think I've come to terms with it now—it's not worth it anymore! I'm going to leave him.

She starts to cry again.

I've been abandoned, I feel so alone. It's very hard Madame . . . it's hard to feel useless. He makes all the important decisions concerning our home with my co-wife. This girl is very young compared to me. My husband could have respected the rules of seniority, but he doesn't care, he regularly berates me in front of her.[3] And when they have problems between them, they work things out in private. I feel like they've joined forces against me. . . . When a problem arises at home, they indirectly make it clear that I bring misfortune.

Case Study 2: Halima, 40 Years Old, Two Miscarriages, "Unfulfilled" (*Gazante* [Z])

Up to this point in her life, Halima has known only the disappointment of miscarriages. After a miscarriage in the fourth month when she was 23 and another three months later, Halima still nurtures the dream of one day being a mother. Yet, at the same time she admits that at her age,

You can't really kid yourself. You just cling to the possibility of God's miracles. Many stories report that miracles can happen. I've often been told there are women who have been able to give birth for the first time at the age of 50, even though we all know 50 is also the age of menopause. Often, even at the age of 45, you can't have children anymore.

Halima was nevertheless entrusted with raising a niece and a younger sister aged six and 13, respectively, in order to help her forget her misfortune.

My niece, born a twin, has been living with me since the age of 20 months, which makes me feel better. A lot of people think I gave birth to her. I moved into the neighborhood right after I took her in. She thinks my husband and I are her real parents. My sister, her real mother, also plays along. But for how long?

3. Editor's note: In most polygynous marriages, the first wife expects to be treated as the "mother of the house," or *uwar gida* in Hausa, a status that confers respect and places her alongside her husband as head of household. Women who enter the household after her are subordinate to her.

I've been living with this worry for a year. She's starting to grow . . . . So far, she's made me happy. In a few days, I'll enroll her in school. When the teacher calls on her, she will need to answer to her real father's name. And I'm the one who will have to prepare her to take on this new role. My little sister, I took her in when she turned five. With her, it's clear I'm not pretending to be her mom. . . . Despite the presence of these two little girls, I really feel alone sometimes. I feel other people's eyes behind my back. I'm often asked, "So, what are you waiting for?" by people I haven't seen in a long time. This question . . . you see, I dread it very much, but it's hard to escape it.

Her married life, which she did not want to talk about at first, is,

almost a nightmare. . . . After 15 months of marriage, my husband quickly took a new wife under pressure from his mother and maternal uncle. At first, he was against the idea. He opposed it without much success. The first year, overall, everything went well. But six months after the birth of my co-wife's first child, a boy, my husband began to change. Sometimes he skips my turns [as sexual partner] in favor of the other. Sometimes, even when he comes to me, we just look at each other. Often, nothing happens between us for several weeks or even months. We fought a lot about the turns, but in the end, I gave up. I preferred to leave him with his conscience. I avoid having conflicts with my co-wife as much as possible, since almost everything turns back against me. She's the *woy kwasa* ("the favorite wife" [Z]).[4] And she delights in letting the whole neighborhood know that our husband neglects me. Do you understand the shame? When she gets started on one of her rants, I hide in my room. . . . I've been through nine years of this hell. After all this, it seems like our husband is taking pity on me and starting to spare me a little. My co-wife is also beginning to calm down a bit now. But that doesn't stop her from provoking me from time to time. Until recently, I wasn't even allowed to assign tasks to one of her children. It's a good thing my sister and niece are here. The few times I've wanted to call for her children it was because those two weren't in the house. Do you know what she'd say to me? "Aren't you a woman? Why bother other people's children? Make one yourself." My husband didn't say things like that to my face, but he'd watch without saying anything. If things are starting to change a little bit, it's certainly due to age. The three of us aren't young anymore.

4. Editor's note: Despite the Islamic injunction to treat all wives equally, local languages reveal the near impossibility of meeting that requirement. In Hausa as well there are words for favorite wife (*mowa*) and unfavored wife (*bora*).

In order to ward off her misfortune, Halima has not been passive. She says she has tried everything, exploring all the spheres of care: traditional, popular, modern.

> For almost 15 years I've almost consulted marabouts exclusively. In fact, even if I give up on everything else, I'll continue the *irkoy nwarey* ("prayers to God" [Z]). I can go two or three months without going to see a marabout but no more than that; I always go back. I saw a lot of traditional healers in Tera and in Dogondoutchi.[5] I even made sacrifices at the foot of the magic stone. In the health centers, they recommended all kinds of treatments. But I refused to have any operation. I've been told that the operation can cause even more problems.[6] I opted to just take the products they prescribed, unreasonably expensive products. I've changed doctors four times. Every time, they tell you "the operation is the ultimate solution." I've asked about seven women who have had the surgery. None of them has had a child so far. . . . In any case, I've looked for all kinds of treatment and at one point I had almost nothing in my room. I'd sold everything that was valuable to be able to cover the costs. I didn't have any jewelry left. There are healers who often asked me for 100,000 CFA francs in one go, promising immediate success. I've been waiting for this miracle for years. For the past three years, I've been doing a bit of business. I gradually replaced what I sold. Now I'm 40 years old and I limit myself to only giving money to marabouts; I've given up on the rest, at least for now.

Case Study 3: Lobbo, 32 Years Old, Never Conceived, "Less of a Woman, Without Children"

At the time of our interview, Lobbo was 32 and lived with two co-wives aged 40 and 28, respectively. Her husband was 49. Like Halima, Lobbo confided that she does not feel like a woman. She, who has not yet given birth to a child, has the feeling of,

> living at the margins of the world of women. I've always had this impression judging from the looks of others. Some people seem compassionate toward me, my fate. Others are very critical and always try to provoke me and challenge

5. Editor's note: Dogondoutchi (in the Hausa Maouri region) and Tera (in the Zarma-Songhay area) are places where highly regarded priest healers continue local spirit mediation despite the rise of Muslim fundamentalism.
6. Editor's note: She may be referring to tuboplasty to clear a blockage of the fallopian tubes. It is the most common treatment for female sterility in Niger and costs nearly the annual salary of a teacher.

me to become pregnant within timelines they choose. Still others are hypocritical. . . . People who live in my circumstances generally end up alone. You're abandoned, first by your husband, then by much of your family. Only people who pity you would think of entrusting their child to you. But that only solves your problem temporarily. At the first opportunity, and if there's any disagreement, the child or their parents will remind you that you are a recipient of their charity, that motherhood is something unknown to you, that you're simply *incapable*. I know what I'm talking about because this happened to a friend of my aunt.

Married for 14 years, Lobbo says she hasn't even experienced a miscarriage, which at least for a moment gives women in her situation some reassurance of their status of a fertile woman:

if I'd had even one miscarriage, I would feel a little like a woman, that is, fertile. Because when you've already "shed one belly," you always hope to "get" another.[7] I've never experienced a late period. When other people, friends, relatives, or neighbors talk about issues surrounding childbirth, I feel embarrassed, lost, and humiliated. So I always try to avoid this type of discussion.

Unlike the women discussed above, Lobbo told me that she has had the help of her husband and some of her in-laws (with the exception of her mother-in-law). Her husband, despite the presence of his two other wives, sometimes accompanies her through parts of her treatment.

Only my mother-in-law doesn't want to see me. It seems I'm an unnecessary burden for her son, who already has a fairly large family of seven children. "God has already blessed him," she would say. And because of this, he should no longer take care of me. Besides, without me, she claims, he would've taken better care of her. My mother-in-law thinks that if my husband is still interested in me despite my problem, it's because I've bewitched him. She even went so far as to see marabouts in order to release him from my enchantment. Because of this kind of thing, I've had to leave our shared home twice. She pressured my husband to separate from me. But it didn't work.

Will it last? I don't know, because she insists on creating conflict in our relationship. You know . . . mothers usually win in this kind of scheming because they're the main point of reference for their sons. My mother-in-law's grip on

7. In local semiology, one says "get the belly" or "make the belly" (*gunde sanbuyan* or *gunde teeyan* in Zarma and *yin ciki* in Hausa) to refer to the state of pregnancy and a "ruined belly" or "to shed the belly" (*gunde hasaraw* or *gunde mun yan* in Zarma and *zubda ciki* in Hausa) for a miscarriage.

her son isn't strong enough yet. The day where she becomes stronger than him (*hane kan a hina* [Z]), I'll have to leave this house, even though I love my husband. When she comes to our house, she makes sure to greet my co-wives first before giving me a dry "hello." When my turn comes, she invents an illness, an errand, something to keep her son away from me. Once, she even blackmailed my husband to repudiate me. Fortunately, that didn't work. . . .

I'm unable to give birth to a child the same way I was born. I won't taste the joy of a successful parent happy who leaves their seed [*dumi* (Z)] when they die. So I am in danger of dying without leaving anyone behind, and that's a real tragedy. It's important to leave your seed behind you, otherwise you'll be forgotten even before you die. You must not die without leaving *dumi*, otherwise you'll be faced with a great catastrophe in your life (*boro ma si bu a mana dumi dirga nan da manti yadin a di andunya fitina* [Z]). My husband thinks I'll have a child eventually, the doctor too, who says I'm still young. My mother-in-law doesn't even want to see me. She thinks three wives is too many for her son. He's fairly decent to me. But he often reminds me of my inability to give him a child. I spend whole nights crying in my room. There's no one to console you. Even my husband, who encourages me to continue treatment, doesn't do anything when he sees me in this state. Instead, it seems that it annoys him. . . .

I still continue the treatments. I go to the health center. They say I don't ovulate, but that the rest of my body is normal. They prescribe me medications. I also see marabouts. Because of religion, my husband doesn't want to hear about traditional healers. So I don't see them. It was suggested that I do a *bori* ceremony. I wanted to do it in secret, but I ended up backing out. I finally realized that what God doesn't give you, you won't get from spirits.[8] My mother recently brought in a marabout from Zinder to take care of me for three months. It costs a lot of money. I don't know if my husband will agree to help me again. It seems this marabout has healed three women.

*****

The stories of Fanta, Halima, and Lobbo suggest that all three women are sterile. In the category of childless women, sterile women seem the most numerous according to medical sources but also in light of my observations made around and inside health centers. The woman who has never known motherhood is, in a way, like a bird that cannot fly. The sterile woman's

---

8. Lobbo's aunt told me that she has taken Lobbo to see healer priests several times herself.

womb, as Lobbo told me, is seen as a "food reserve." Consequently, Lobbo can only accommodate and "enjoy" the prolificacy of others. Some people remind her that she is only on the "margins of womanhood." Women who have never conceived are ignorant of its mysteries. If these women are to be believed, the secrets of conception are immense; and experiencing even a small part of it puts one in a more favorable position.

The stories presented here highlight the issue of intergenerational transmission. Being able to contribute to the continuity of the family line appears to be crucial in the construction of one's identity. In numerous interviews the breakdown of family perpetuation occurs in at least two forms: breakdown in the transmission of a family's memory through its name and breakdown in the transmission of property. In the first form of discontinuity, the sterile individual bears the responsibility for having interrupted one of life's cycles. Female infertility, as Philippe Bessoles (2001) puts it, is evidence of the "breakdown of the ascending lineage with the failure of the descending lineage" (p. 108). The sterile person breaks, in spite of herself, a vital chain that is meant to unfold indefinitely through time. With this rift, she interrupts to some extent the continuation of the family memory. Beyond the loss of the patronym, which perpetuates their husband's line, women fear the failure of any pronouncement of their own name.[9]

> If you don't leave a child behind, you're easily forgotten. No one will remember for very long that you existed on Earth. They'll forget everything, including your name. (Madame HZ2, 42 years old, childless, Kirkissoye district)

In Chapter 1, I discussed a strong association that is made between sterility and death. It is all the more significant that my respondents put forward the idea that a person who dies without leaving descendants has never existed. As one childless 47-year-old man told me, "In people's minds, if you die childless, it's like you never existed. Even living, you mean very little to people; even more so when you die" (JK, welder, Kalley-Est district).

Reproduction also makes possible the transmission of a material (wealth) or political (aristocratic title) inheritance. The transmission of

---

9. Editor's note: Many mothers in Niger are referred to less by their own formal names than through teknonyms. Thus, Halima, a woman married to Mahamane, might be referred to as "mother of Abdou," rather than Madame Mahamane. Abdou might be referred to as "son of Halima" or as "son of Mahamane." In a sense, the boy child's existence gives regular reference to her own existence. In establishing social relations, Abdou will invoke Halima regularly long after her death whenever he establishes his own position in extended family networks.

a title to one's descendants is related, but not identical, to the question of name transmission. Everyone has a name to convey, but not everyone has an aristocratic rank to defend and safeguard. Any breakdown in the transmission of property is a particular concern for those who are wealthy. Men, as well as women, care about the transmission of their heritage when they die. No one can tolerate the absence of heirs because it reflects a double loss: of child and of fortune. The idea of leaving your inheritance to anyone other than your own children appears intolerable. One woman in the Terminus district, Madame MG, who is 43 years old and childless, explained the following to me:

> In dying, it would be best if your property were inherited by a part of you, that is, your children. But without children, it's in some cases the husband, parents, or siblings who will "eat" your belongings (*I ga ni almano nwa* [Z]). What's more, even total strangers might inherit from you. And there you've doubly lost. If you die knowing your child succeeds you in the management of your property, you've lived a truly fulfilled life.

For most sterile people, the impossibility of being an ancestor is all-consuming. In Cameroon, as Christine Tichit (2009) writes, beyond social recognition in daily life, "to have no descendants is to be condemned to the impossibility of becoming an ancestor and therefore to disappear from the memory of the living" (p. 6). The search to become an ancestor stems from a deep need to accomplish a kind of "extension ad extra" of one's being through the birth of a child (Erny 1988: 21). Women without children live the almost daily anguish of not perpetuating filial ties because "creating a child is above all creating time" or "giving life is first of all giving one's life," writes Philippe Bessoles (2001: 111). The discontinuity of the self is closely linked to familial discontinuity, but it is experienced by the sterile individual in a much more poignant way. The discontinuity of the self necessarily implies a loss of the self because, more than simply wanting a child, the sterile woman seeks, as Marie Santiago-Delafosse puts it, "a part of herself" (1995: 168). To cite Madame MG again,

> I'm in danger of dying without leaving anyone behind, and that's a real tragedy. When you're remembered after your death, it's because you left someone, and they'll say, "that's so and so's son, so and so's daughter." But if you've never had a child, who'll think of you? No one, Madame! Whether they behave well or not, people will say "there are so and so's children." You're present in people's minds. But if you live alone and you die alone, it's different.

THE LOSS OF YOUNG CHILDREN: FORGOTTEN FERTILITY

Case Study 4: Fadima, 41 Years Old, Two Children Who Died in Infancy, "I Feel Deeply Unhappy"

I had my first child 18 years ago. He was born premature at seven months. For the first three months, we had to stay in either the maternity ward or the hospital. Many people thought he was going to die even before the baptism. But he held on for four and a half more months. When he died, he weighed no more than three kilos. Ten months later, I was pregnant again, after which I gave birth to a little girl who was taken away by measles when she was only six months old. I've been waiting desperately for a pregnancy for about 15 years. I haven't even had a miscarriage since then. It's so strange. I consulted everyone: the herbal healers, the traditional healers, the marabouts, and especially the Central Maternity Hospital and the hospital. I've paid for exorbitantly priced medications. Most recently, they wanted to operate on me. But at my age, 41, it's very risky. And I think I'm going to make up my mind: I have to learn to forget these things. . . .

My friends who gave birth for the first time at the same time as me already have grandchildren. They've seen their children grow up, get married, and multiply, and I saw mine die. I buried them instead of them giving me a funeral with dignity. . . . My husband celebrated a second marriage with a 17-year-old girl. If my children were alive, they'd be older than her. Long before she was with us, my husband stopped providing for my minor needs: clothing, pocket money. . . . The only thing I haven't been deprived of yet is food. We are not short on food in my family. My family isn't poor. . . .

People who have been in my situation and who have found success have told me about great healers from Burkina Faso, who I went to see right away. I had to go there several times. But nothing worked. This is certainly the destiny that God has reserved for me. I have no choice but to accept it. This is my sad fate! . . . When my friends talk about their children, I feel deeply unhappy; I relive the times when I was pregnant, the times when my children left me. In short, I see the whole movie of my life as an empty woman, an unhappy woman, a lonely woman. No matter how much love your husband has for you, if you don't have someone to call you "mommy," you're very lonely. Filial love is eternal, while all the rest is a hoax.

My first co-wife died in childbirth three years ago. I don't have a new co-wife yet, but I do know that my husband has relationships outside the home. Recently, he made someone pregnant. He hasn't told me yet, but I know he'll soon be marrying the girl he got pregnant. It would be the logical next step. My husband has always been discreet about my disadvantage, but his family talks about it nonstop. His sisters and aunts are unbearable. They're often very unpleasant to me. So are my husband's sisters-in-law.

For the past year, Fadima has not taken any steps to treat her condition. She says she now puts her trust in God:

Many people have never seen a doctor, a marabout, or a healer to have children. It was God who took care of their fate. So why wouldn't he take care of mine? Human beings are often impatient. That's why I'm waiting for a sign from God now. After all, it's he who decides to create and destroy. I never forget to pray to him. As they say, it's better to deal with God than with his prophets. I've spent a lot on marabouts and healers. Now I prefer to speak directly to him so he can hear me better and quickly.

But she finishes her speech without the slightest conviction:

but who knows, if there's someone who's sure to work, maybe I'll go and see him. I have no *dumi* ("progeny" [Z]).[10] When I think about it today, I would've much preferred to have died before my children; it's certain that I'd always be remembered through them. A child allows you to exist even after you die.

Case Study 5: Fennye, 43 Years Old, Two Children Who Died in Infancy, "the Open Grave"

Fennye buys and resells various products such as incense, clothing, and cosmetics. This activity earns her enough money to provide for herself and take care of her family (her father, mother, and two little brothers). She gave birth to two children, each of whom died before the age of one. The first, she says, died mysteriously at two months, and the second died of a respiratory infection. She has been desperately seeking to have children for 11 years. Now, at the age of 43, she has less and less hope and continually asks herself,

What did I do to God that was so horrible he should deprive me of the most important thing on earth? I find my life meaningless because I haven't personally given life. Based on what I have experienced, a woman's life is of value only when she herself has given birth one or more times. For this reason, my death will also have no meaning. Do you know that even after death, man continues to live? That's why relatives of the deceased always take care to cover his grave so he never lacks shade. This shade is provided with wet or dry branches usually coming from thorny trees that can prevent animals from reaching the grave. This is why those in the east [of Niger] call an open grave "a grave that is thornless."

10. The term *dumi* is polysemic and signifies species, kinship, ethnicity, race, and seed in Zarma. In this context, the term can be translated as "progeny." *Iri* (seed or kind) is the Hausa equivalent of *dumi*.

That's how I think of myself personally. Neither of my two children survived more than four months. As far as many people are concerned, especially those who live far from me, I've never been a mother. In a way, they're right. They've never seen me pregnant or in labor, let alone with a baby on my back. If I die like this, that is, without children, who will mourn me? No one, or close to that. My family will for the first few days, but you're soon forgotten. . . . My husband already had four children with his late wife. If he keeps me at home, it's more so I can take care of them, and anyway he doesn't want any more. He also keeps me a little out of pity. It's not because he loves me that he keeps me by his side. He's getting older (61) and can no longer afford to care for another woman. I've been taking care of myself for a long time. In the end, it doesn't cost him anything to keep me in his home. His family insisted that he remarry, but he objected. Before he retired, some even asked that he repudiate me. There, too, they haven't yet been successful. From this point of view, I can say that I'm a little lucky compared to some women, because they've had multiple husbands deluding themselves that they might get pregnant.

Fennye has tried every possible treatment to ward off evil. She has also made two trips to Nigeria to see a prominent marabout and a famous traditional healer. In her quest for treatment, she estimates that she has spent more than one million CFA francs.[11] With each of these trips, she said, her husband was content to send her off with a quick "Good luck!" She ends her story with a smirk. In questioning her sad fate, she takes refuge behind her dark and sarcastic sense of humor: "I, the empty gourd, sadly empty, why am I hopelessly empty? When will I finally be full? I hope it'll be before the hen grows its teeth, otherwise. . . ." She conveys the drama of her life through self-mockery.

*****

Fadima and Fennye have experienced pregnancy, childbirth, breastfeeding—aspects of motherhood—but the early loss of their children seems to negate their status as fertile women. The maternal role they played is erased from the memories of those who surround them. Due to childhood illnesses and malnutrition, many women in Niger lose their babies within the first few weeks or months of giving birth. Such infants do not yet have social personhood. In Niger, those who die before

11. Editor's note: CFA is the monetrary unit of the African Financial Community of West African States. In 2006 one million CFA would have been roughly $1,950.

the fortieth day after childbirth are not considered to be dead but rather "returned"; it is considered that they have "left" or that they "did not stay." There is little sadness regarding their fate. But the disappointed mother will secretly fear that this child may be her last.

When the infant has survived beyond this pivotal period, it has begun to be socialized—it is more fully a person. Fadima and Fennye both experienced a fleeting happiness that has been erased from the memories of their respective families. They witnessed their pregnancies. Some watched them give birth, and others saw them as mothers carrying their children. Though they did accomplish what Camille Lacoste-Dujardin ([1985] 1996: 116) calls the "procreative patrilineal service," the impossibility of marking their maternity in the long term places them today in roughly the same position as those who still seek conception and procreation. As Fennye said, to no longer and never again hear herself be called "Mommy" deprives a woman of peace of mind.

SUBFERTILITY: A SHORT REPRODUCTIVE CAREER

Case Study 6: Gooro, 38 Years Old, Mother of One Child, "It's Like Being Half Naked"

Gooro had her first pregnancy in 1983 while she was a student in the fourth year.[12] Abandoned by her boyfriend who did not recognize the child as his own, she nevertheless managed to finish her studies brilliantly. Today, she earns a good living with an "interesting" job in a government ministry. In 1989, she married a civil servant from the same ministry who was already married to a woman with two children. Gooro recounts her life:

At first, everything went well between my co-wife and me, between my husband and me. This idyll lasted two and a half years. My delay in conceiving was not a problem for my husband. Since I had already given birth to a boy, there was no doubt in his mind that I could conceive again. To support me, he even agreed to welcome my child under his roof. . . . After the third year, my husband was no longer the same. Under the pretext of a disagreement between his children and my son, he sent the boy to live with my parents. Then he accused me of having led a debauched life in the past, before and after the birth of my child. He claims

12. Editor's note: Equivalent to the penultimate year of courses before students enter high school; students in *classe de 4ème* are generally about 13–15 years of age.

I used contraception to run after many men, which isn't true. My first boyfriend disappointed me so much I went three years without another attachment. The first relationship I agreed to after this disappointment was with him, my current husband.

There are experiences in life that teach you lessons. I understood that very early. Out of love, I gave myself to a boy from my school when I was barely 16 years old. This boy, for fear of commitment, abandoned me when I needed him the most. You see, I could no longer trust men. . . . The clinical examinations to detect my problems didn't reveal anything serious. Everything is normal with me. The marabouts told me it was my co-wife's fault—that she'd "tied" me. That she'd sworn not to give me the chance to give heirs to my husband who, I remind you, has a small fortune. Many clairvoyants and healers have told me that I could have children by remarrying. After the father of my child, my husband is the only one I've loved and still love. I've never been able to leave him, even if he doesn't care about me at all anymore. . . .

I often hide my child for fear of being further insulted. A child out of wedlock is very dishonorable in our circles. . . . My son is now 21, but I don't feel fulfilled at all. With only one child, you're never at peace. I live with constant stress. I'm always afraid something will happen to him. It's like if you only have one shirt—if you lose it, you'll be naked. I'm already poorly clothed, and I fear becoming naked. Having only one child is like being half-naked. . . . At the Central Maternity Hospital, I was told that everything seems normal. The doctor told me I need to do more tests. I'm waiting for the end of the treatment he gave me.

While telling her story, Gooro's drawn face was at once melancholy and distant.

*****

For various reasons, some women fail to give birth to more than one or two children and are stricken with what is referred to medically as "secondary infertility" or subfertility. This is the case for Gooro who, although she has given birth to one child, feels no more fulfilled than a sterile woman. In pro-natalist Niger, not only procreation but repeated procreation is socially prescribed. Having one or two children does not appear to satisfy the majority of those who I interviewed. Subfertile women who have had one or two births are commonly perceived as sterile. They are characterized by others as "infertile," "unfortunate," or "afraid."

"A Subfertile Woman Is Basically a Childless Woman"

Gooro told me that, "a woman who has only knelt to give birth once in her life, whether the child is alive or not; we can't say she was truly a mother."[13] Gooro continued that a woman who has one child,

> just had the chance to take a glimpse at the life of a mother (*a zonkom nya kaloora hinne no* [Z]). She still has a long way to go, just as a woman who has never given birth does in order to take pride in herself for being a mother in society. I say this because people have told me this indirectly several times, and it's not untrue.

Having numerous children is incredibly important. In rural areas, the size of a family determines its labor force and therefore its productivity. In the city, the precariousness of employment and the high cost of living, among other constraints, would seem to run counter to this strategy. Nevertheless, deeply engrained values such as the desire for the social prestige associated with the ideal of the "big family" still encourage men and women to widen their family circle. In Niger's big cities, and Niamey in particular, the "big family" enables family members to benefit from large numbers. Here, the social value linked to fertility reaches beyond the individual or conjugal framework. Wedding and funeral announcements through media such as radio and print publicize the prestige of such families.[14]

"A Subfertile Woman Is Considered to Be Fearful"

A woman's first delivery constitutes a significant physical, physiological, and psychological metamorphosis. It is a moment that marks adulthood and signifies the conversion of a girl to a woman. This metamorphosis is accompanied by danger and anxiety, often linked in local thinking to the Abrahamic tradition attributing the pain of childbirth to punishment for human sin (Genesis 3:16). Adrienne Rich suggestively observes in *Of Woman Born* that, "Women who refuse to become mothers are not merely emotionally suspect, but are dangerous. Not only do they refuse to continue the species; they also deprive society of its emotional leaven—the suffering of the mother" (1995: 169).

---

13. Women in Niger have long given birth on their hands and knees, and continue to do so outside of healthcare structures.

14. Editor's note: Such announcements entail the reading of long lists of the names of individuals and households related to the relevant parties.

The failure of a woman to face the pain of childbirth is judged harshly in Niger. There is a perception that, for some women, the physical aftereffects of childbirth manifest themselves in what might be called "maternophobia," a kind of psychological inhibition regarding childbearing. This is why, in certain representations, those who suffer from sterility are considered responsible for their condition due to a refusal to suffer the pain of childbirth. Whether accurate or not, it is said that echoes of the pain of childbirth reached them and conditioned them to "unconsciously lock" their bodies (cf. Deutsch [1949] 1987: 99).

"A Subfertile Woman Is an 'Unlucky' Woman"

It is believed that the subfertile woman faces misfortune. Though she is not completely unlucky like the sterile woman, one cannot say that she is fortunate. The fear of losing an only child haunts subfertile women. As SH, a 37-year-old married man with one child, told me, "A woman who has only one child, for example, is neither unlucky nor truly lucky. She's in between (*Manti bon futu no amma i si ne mo bon kaana no* [Z])" (Karradjé district). And, as Gooro put it above, "With only one child, you're never at peace. I live with constant stress. I'm always afraid something will happen to him." The maternal happiness of a subfertile woman (generally a woman with one child) is considered to be "unclear" both by those concerned and by others. As 47-year-old AO with six children said to me, "What I say isn't mean, it's a very common idea: a subfertile woman is perceived as a *bon futu* ("unlucky woman" [Z]). You, me, everyone believes it" (Gaweye district).

IMPERILED WOMANHOOD

What conclusions can be drawn from these six stories? Women who have never conceived, those who lost their children at a young age, and subfertile women are generally considered by society to be in the same situation. For the three categories of women presented above, the absence of children is synonymous with discontinuity, both familial and individual. In Nigerien society, giving birth to a child who survives and who becomes an adult is the real guarantee of one's social advancement. Paola Tabet argues that the asymmetry of the sexual division of labor "must be analyzed as a political relationship between the sexes" (1998: 15) best approached through the actual instruments men and women use in production. But here I will approach women's gender identity through the question of how a woman's lack of children impacts her social identity.

The quest for identity among women rests upon their reproductive capacities. The construction of a woman's identity involves a complex process where emotional, intellectual, and biological capacities are based on childbirth. Childbirth transforms a woman's body and identity. The aspect of womanly identity represented by motherhood takes on a sacred character. The interdependence of womanhood and maternity exposes an infertile woman to a life of fear of being beholden to society for a debt that she cannot repay. This sense of inadequacy is symptomatic of women who have never given birth as well as those whose progeny is deemed inadequate.

Many of the women I encountered yielded to others' perceptions of them. The women I interviewed connect womanhood (*woyborotaray* [Z]) to a variety of signs such as menstruation, breasts, childbirth, and mothering (see also Journet 1985: 27; Héritier 1996).[15] Given the significance of motherhood to the concepts of femininity and womanhood, many women said such things as, "I don't feel like a woman" or "I'm unfulfilled." Women experienced infertility and subfertility as a crisis of adulthood and identity. They have not experienced the empowerment of becoming fully adult. They feel that they have not yet mourned the end of their childhood or their adolescence. Bringing one or more children into the world enables one to get one's bearings in a new world (that of adult parents) and to take permanent leave of another. The simple fact of being married does not automatically break the chains that bind the individual to this period of her life. It is through a fertile marriage that the adult woman is truly emancipated.

Having a manly or womanly identity brings a sense of balance to the individual. Lacking this balance contributes to a weakening of ties or a heightened complexity in an individual's relationships with the rest of society. As we have seen, women struggling with fertility fear or avoid interacting with others because such interactions can be humiliating and demeaning. Women and men in other places, especially in the West, have been able to pursue alternative models to fulfillment and a socially enhanced life without children. A sense of value resulting from such models of full adulthood softens the blow of childlessness, making it easier to accept and accommodate infertility. Through work, reputation, wealth, and power, individuals who have—sometimes voluntarily—renounced motherhood or fatherhood can attain a sense of social achievement. Investing in

15. Editor's note: In many languages, the same word can mean "woman" or "wife." In Zarma *weyboro* can mean "female person," "woman," or "wife."

professional success, however, may also be seen by others as self-centered. An upward professional trajectory often causes a delay in marriage and childbearing for women, for motherhood can be an obstacle to professional advancement. Sometimes as a result, pursuing a career compromises a woman's childbearing ability. Some of these women are not childless by choice but adapt to the decline in fertility with age and life without children.

By contrast, in Niamey, sterility and subfertility undermine a woman's sense of her own identity as a woman. Societal exclusion prompts many women to pursue strategies for social reinstatement by earning family recognition first. This family recognition primarily involves fostering children. The majority of my respondents also sought to improve their social standing through commerce, a profession, political commitments, or involvement in civil society associations. All these attempts by infertile women to counter their social marginality do not fundamentally change the negative evaluations of others because these successes are not recognized as legitimate alternatives to motherhood.

Of the women I met, only three stated firmly that their investment outside the maternal framework has satisfied them. Hadjia F. is one of them. Hadjia F., 53 years old, has never had children. She does not complain much:

> I raised three foster children—two girls and a boy. The two girls have already married. With my activities, I earn enough money and I believe today I can say *Alhamdulillah* [Ar. "Praise be to God"] even if I didn't give birth myself. I used to see life too negatively. But that's no longer the case today. I went to Mecca to do my pilgrimage twice. I think I'll still take two or three children under my protection. At this age, we have to forget about what they call motherhood.

Hadjia F. shares the condition of childlessness with the other women we have seen so far, but she has followed a socio-professional trajectory that many of her peers have not. The first wife of an important politician, she has significant economic capital at her disposal. She has invested much into her husband's party, which earned her a political position. She held this position for three years, which opened other prospects for her. Hadjia F. has in turn built up a social and political clientele who show her respect and loyalty.[16]

---

16. Editor's note: She has also marked her success in life through the attainment of the title *Hadjia*, which affirms her identity as a devout Muslim woman. For an example of a woman, Malama A'ishatu Hamani Zarmakoy Dancandu, who "used to cry for not having children" and found happiness and purpose when she completed her Qu'ranic training, see Alidou (2005: 54–55).

Women like Hadjia F. are rare. Most Nigerien women have fewer opportunities than Hadjia F., which means that motherhood takes precedence over any other arena of social success. As one housewife, 29-year-old Madame MA, told me, "Even if you're offered the whole world, you'll still suffer from having no children. Deep down, you represent nothing" (co-wife of Madame HZ2, three children, Kirkissoye district). For women, giving life is synonymous with good fortune, social achievement, and an infinite and fulfilled life. Infertile women are often left to fend for themselves, leading a lonely fight because of, as one teacher put it, "the blame for sterility placed on the woman and the advantages that polygamy grants to men." This asymmetry in the imputation of infertility, argues Françoise Héritier (1984), results from a societal desire to maintain a sexual hierarchy. This asymmetry marginalizes women, which in turn incites their desperate quests for treatment.

CHAPTER 4
The Emotional Weight of Childlessness

Childless women experience a broad array of emotions over their reproductive careers (joy, guilt, affection, shame, doubt, despair, anticipation, loneliness). For sterile women conflicting feelings can follow one after another. Women facing infertility or subfertility also confront a range of moral questions. I had not originally set out to analyze these feelings and moral quandaries, but they imposed themselves on me as the research progressed.

An anthropological analysis of affect or *sensibilités* can be useful in understanding the experiences of infertile women. Out of this new approach, which psychologizes anthropology, or conversely anthropologizes psychology, I have been inspired by the innovative work of Yannick Jaffré (2003b, 2003c, 2003d), who urges a renewal of attention to emotions in the field of anthropology of health. Historians such as Arlette Farge (1997), Alain Corbin (1991), Lucien Febvre (1992), Jacques Revel (1996), and Michel de Certeau (1990), to name a few, have greatly influenced scholarship on emotion. Febvre defines the French word *sensibilité* as "affective life and its manifestations," the study of which he argues should be central to the work of historians (1992: 222).

An anthropology of emotions must address an individual's historical milieu (Revel 1996). Thus, the suffering of a woman seeking to bear a child or treatment to ward off bad luck or simply fate has to be situated within her historical context. Emotions are not to be understood simply as physiological or irrational by-products; they deserve attention from the anthropologist. We should analyze emotions to better understand the aspects of cognition and behavior that are hidden from ordinary audiences (Jaffré 2003c). Here, I seek not to practice psychology but to

Yearning and Refusal. Hadiza Moussa, Edited by Alice J. Kang and Barbara M. Cooper, Oxford University Press.
© Oxford University Press 2023. DOI: 10.1093/oso/9780197662113.003.0005

analyze how emotions are socially and historically constructed and to understand how emotions influence the social trajectories and choices made by individuals.

What types of emotional struggles do infertile women in Niger experience? How does infertility disrupt their imagining of the future? What imbalances are created within the close family sphere—that is, the conjugal sphere—and within the extended family circle? How do infertile women organize or reorganize their emotional universes to accommodate or adapt to a "new" identity or to an identity "reshaped" by the eyes of others? The aim here is to draw out the experiences and feelings of infertile women and to analyze the suffering linked to their *manque d'enfant* (absence of children). I will take up the emotional suffering, guilt, shame, confidence, hope, and despair that punctuate their reflections as well as how these feelings are socially constructed. I take up a semantic exploration of the language they employ to discuss their feelings. This will also enable us to understand how women internalize and appropriate the dominant social norms of Nigerien society in their relationships with themselves and with others. First, however, I will address some of the difficulties inherent in the analysis of emotions.

OBSTACLES TO THE STUDY OF EMOTION

Identifying and analyzing emotions are difficult. Since emotions have no objective external form, as Jaffré points out, "the question arises as to what material the observation of feelings, which are never presented except as 'signifieds', might rest upon" (2003a: 66). The same author specifies, "This is why painting a picture—even making a sketch . . .—of the feelings one experiences involves reflection upon a subjectivity and an interiority that can only be spoken in half-words, or evoked, or taken by surprise in the course of daily activities" (2003a: 66). The challenge of scientifically deciphering emotions is also due to the multiplicity and sometimes to the ambivalence of feelings that overlap with each other. After citing joy and sadness, feelings of the ego, love and hate, fear and hope as constituting the fundamental feelings of human beings, Jean Maisonneuve illustrates the analogies that exist between them:

> It goes without saying that there are intimate affinities between several of these feelings: pleasure normally calls for joy, which inclines to love and to hope; this is the realm of fulfillment, of communion, of trust; in a word, the realm of "yes." Conversely, pain calls for sadness, which inclines to hatred, worry

and despair: this is the realm of refusal, isolation, mistrust, the realm of "no."
(1993: 50)

Like love, emotions such as hope, shame, doubt, joy, faith, loneliness, sadness, and guilt, to name a few, all are subjects of study that are necessarily elusive in the human sciences. Jaffré, recognizing the pitfalls facing the researcher analyzing people's emotional and moral lives, writes, "in the absence of a shared means of measuring emotion, when we describe what we imagine another is experiencing, we never know whether that emotion is projected improperly upon him, or whether we wrongly withhold the attribution of different emotion from him" (2003a: 66). Emotions are linked to codes, to internal or, in fact, internalized experiences that are difficult to decipher through the typical forms of anthropological analysis. Nevertheless, a study focused on feelings may reveal important and overlooked aspects of the social and individual experience.

The analysis of feelings, *sensibilités*, or emotions can lead to an impasse: translating "emic" terms into "etic" concepts. Lay and learned categories, when they are examined in isolation, are vague concepts with meanings and significations that interfere with one another (Ouattara 1999). The semantic variations of a single term are therefore just as complex as their transcription from one language to another. Not surprisingly, it is difficult to arrive at a uniform definition that can be agreed upon even within a group that shares the same sociocultural referents.

THE ABSENCE OF CHILDREN AND THE ABSENCE OF AFFECTION

Infertility in women, this "emptiness," is the basis of great emotional misery and is itself the source of marital instability. The affection a husband and wife have for one another, no matter its intensity, generally dissolves in the absence of children. "Children give birth to love in a couple or strengthen it when it already exists" is a phrase both mothers and non-mothers uttered repeatedly during our conversations. Many of the women I interviewed repeated the same expression: "a birth enhances marriage" (*hayyon a ga hijay kaanandi* [Z] and *aihuwa na kyautada aure* [H]). After the announcement of a pregnancy, feelings of affection and love strengthen in the conjugal realm. As numerous examples attest, the arrival of a child in the household creates a brand new and strong emotional atmosphere:

> When my co-wife got pregnant, my husband was in her room all the time. He seemed very happy. He would often leave his workplace and come just

to inquire about my co-wife's condition. He brought her all kinds of small gifts: good food, perfume, etc. When his family came to visit, he only talked about her. Polygamous life should require him to be a little discreet about his feelings, but he hardly hides them. My co-wife lived a double, even triple happiness: the pregnancy, the love and preference of our husband, and the consideration of our in-laws. And I'm there too, more and more unhappy. (Fanta, Case Study 1)

Giving birth creates new feelings, even if in some cases they are ephemeral, especially when many children are born into a home. However, these happy feelings are not inevitable. There are other situations in which a man turns his back on his wife who has just become pregnant. This is most often linked to the physical changes that modify the woman's relationship to sex as a pregnancy progresses.

And yet, the first experience of childbirth always seems exceptional. For the young couple, the first childbirth marks a transition, more pleasurable than the end of adolescence that comes with bodily maturity. After the rituals performed during childhood, which require circumcision for boys and sometimes excision for girls, marriage and parenthood are the major moments of transition that occur in the achievement of adulthood. For women in particular, this adulthood translates into the fulfillment of conjugal, maternal, and nurturing roles.

Instead of being here to breastfeed, to feed, to nurse (*ay ma zankay taway* [Z]), or educate my children, I'm still trying to mature. When you haven't had a child, you too feel like a child, or at least that's the impression you give a lot of people, starting with your girlfriends who've already given birth. (Madame ZI, 33 years old, childless, woman operated on at the Central Maternity Hospital)

The husband's indifference toward his infertile wife can, in some cases, turn into esteem when she finally succeeds in giving birth to a child, even if in the meantime his other wives may have filled this void in her husband's heart. The example of Madame GS reveals the degree to which the feeling of love is drawn from childbirth.

We got married when I was 19. I stayed 12 years without children. Only once did I have a miscarriage . . . well, I think I did. After my period was seven weeks late, I bled heavily for a week. I was told it was a miscarriage. In any case, I only shed blood. My husband took a second wife two and a half years after our marriage. Right away, she had a boy. After that, she had two more children. My husband really wasn't interested in me. Often, he would refuse my turns to go sleep in my co-wife's room. Even when he spends the night with me, he's always quick to leave. . . . In the thirteenth year of my marriage, I finally became pregnant. It was an indescribable joy for me. . . . My husband became much more attentive toward me—he talks to me more kindly, he gives me gifts to which I wasn't entitled before. Now he asks about my health, he lingers a lot in my room. I think he loves me now. (Madame GS, pregnant with her second child, Lakouroussou district)

LONELINESS THROUGH MULTIPLE FORMS OF EXCLUSION

As Lobbo (Case Study 3) told me, "People in my situation usually end up alone. They abandon you. Your husband first. Then much of your family." Lobbo and many infertile women experience ostracism in multiple spheres of social life: conjugal exclusion, exclusion from the marital "lineage," exclusion from one's own family, social exclusion, and self-exclusion from social circles are all a part of the different forms of "rejection" they face. Loneliness often overwhelms infertile women.

Exclusion in One's Own Marriage

Time and again in this analysis, we have seen how precarious childless marriages can be for women. The following story conveys the lonely life that some infertile women say they lead:

Before his remarriage, my husband would desert the house altogether, and more often, he organized inopportune trips with his friends. As the house was empty, he hardly cared what happened there; he almost never called. The rare times he did were when he'd left behind business and wanted to inquire about its progress. And even when he wasn't traveling, he stayed out. I was almost always alone, except when I had visitors. Once I had a severe attack of malaria, and it was one of our neighbors whose wife is a friend of mine who rushed me to the hospital. . . . There was no way to reach him. He came back late at night. There was no one to tell him; everyone was asleep. He thought I'd run away. And he really didn't care. It was only the next day that the same neighbor came to tell him I was in the hospital. . . . Most of the time, I'm alone. If I had children, he would've paid more attention to me. The proof is that when my co-wife arrived and had children, he was more present at home. (Fanta, Case Study 1)

Exclusion from the Marital Lineage

According to a Kabyle proverb recorded by Camille Lacoste-Dujardin, "The girl is like a swallow under the roof: she's not settled anywhere until she's a fertile mother in the family of another" ([1985] 1996: 116). Similarly, some of my respondents feel marginalized by their in-laws:

> My in-laws are only interested in my co-wife. You get the impression I don't exist. It's mostly the women who behave this way. Whether it's sisters, cousins, aunts, or mother, they're all waiting for me to have my divorce papers. (Fadima, Case Study 4)

> Family members are very involved in a couple's life. In cases of infertility, they can suggest or dictate a divorce—even when the husband is not yet ready for this. They say, for example, "You suffer and waste your time on a sterile person. Go get married." So even when you love your wife, they can separate you. And little by little, without really realizing it, he gravitates away from the person everyone else ignores. An infertile woman—she's separated from her husband; she's separated from the rest of the world. (Madame IM, 43 years old, childless, Balafon district)

The marginalization that the childless woman experiences in the marital lineage becomes more acute when the couple lives in the "big house" together with a large part of the husband's family.[1] The husband, for various reasons, often prefers to live near his family (father, mother, brothers and sisters, etc.). In this kind of residential unit, several households live side by side. Married sisters usually live elsewhere, but many brothers bring their wives into the family concession. These sisters-in-law are called *woycina kongrom* (Z) or *kishiyar samri* or *matar samri* (H),[2] and in many cases the situation provokes stronger jealousy than that between co-wives.

> A woman who has never given birth is never fully integrated into her husband's family. Besides, in some cases, even when she has children, if she isn't from the

1. The "big house" (*hu beero or windi beero* [Z]) is a residence where parents and married children live together. Almost all married women, whether fertile or infertile, prefer not to live in the "big house," particularly in the case of a marriage between close relatives, such as cousins. Women accuse their in-laws of being voyeurs of their conjugal lives even more when everyone lives together in the same residence. The interventionism of in-laws is likely to undermine a household's stability.

2. Editor's note: The Hausa expression emphasizes that the woman, as the wife of a "youth" (*samari* or *saurayi*) who is himself a younger male member of the family, is at the bottom of the household hierarchy.

same family as her husband, she still remains an outsider for many (*nga yaw no* [Z]). (MI, 55, bus driver, Talladjé district)

Being childless subjects a woman to all kinds of challenges including jeers, as pointed out by the following woman, who was undergoing surgery for primary infertility at the Central Maternity Hospital in Niamey:

> Because we live in the big house, my husband was encouraged to remarry. . . . All my sisters-in-law had children. So I often endure taunts and provocations of all kinds from them. They always take the opportunity to put the issue of mother-hood and children at the center of conversations. When our husbands are there, it's often much worse. They definitely want my husband to take stock of our situation: a life without children. It was so incessant he gave in very quickly. I thought I'd be forgotten with the pregnancy of my co-wife; unfortunately, it's gotten worse for me. (Madame FM, 30 years old, childless, teacher, operated on at the Central Maternity Hospital)

The derogatory remarks made by women within the home (whether by sisters-in-law or co-wives) contribute to the othering of the childless woman in patrilineal marriages. In Joola society, as Odile Journet writes, "a woman who has no children occupies a bastard position: excluded from rituals or the main associations of women, she is suspected (and ultimately rejected) by the marital lineage. During fertility celebrations, which are still prac-ticed even in urban areas, she is the subject of slander and of provocations ritually uttered against her" (1991: 20–21). Similarly, among Yorubas in Nigeria, Winny Koster found that "about one-fifth of the women with in-fertility problems had to endure neglect, verbal abuse, and anger, slightly more frequently from their in-laws than from their husbands" (2003: 285).

Exclusion from One's Own Family

Some infertile women experience marginalization from their own relatives. Despite forms of solidarity around the infertile woman, one can detect among members of her family attitudes that contribute to the weakening of her position at home. In the sibling group, those who do not have chil-dren have the least certain standing in the memory of the lineage.

> They call me less and less often for family ceremonies. Some people pretend I'm already dead. They no longer include me in their activities, or rarely do so, even though the whole family gets together for them. They apologize afterward,

pretending to have forgotten me. That may be true. It's really not surprising that a person who's alone might be forgotten. Sometimes my husband, even though I live under the same roof, forgets about me. Sometimes they'll tell me when they're gathering contributions for the celebration, but then I'm left out of everything later. The important questions are handled by those who have already secured the family's future with children. I mean very little to them. (Halima, Case Study 2)

The family discards, whether deliberately or not, those who have not "enriched" it with offspring. Descendants are, depending on the circumstances, asked to participate in the life of the group. In activities of collective interest, families with many children play a decisive role in the decisions and execution of tasks requiring physical energy. During various ceremonies (e.g., baptisms, marriages, funerals), domestic activities are carried out by the entire familial network: brothers, sisters, cousins, and aunts. The preparation of food, cleaning the house, and the oversight of guests are most often left to the youngest ones, with the parents being simple supervisors. An infertile person or a couple without children contributes nothing of significance to the group. Even apart from executing physical tasks, the ability of a family to mobilize its members for a given cause is a source of social validation. In urban centers like Niamey, the ethos of the "big family" remains highly valued despite the emergence of new values linked to the nuclear household.

Infertile individuals are therefore not able to contribute to the family tree and to multiply family relationships between ascendants and descendants, on the one hand, and among descendants, on the other. In the latter case, possible affiliations between the children of brothers and sisters, highly valued in the region, are also forestalled.

Furthermore, at another generational register, grandparents request the assistance of their grandchildren on either a temporary basis to execute certain tasks or on a permanent basis to offer them daily support. Conversely, grandparents may be asked by their children to look after their grandchildren. In this case, the grandchildren return to the place from which their parents came, strengthening filial ties while providing domestic help to their elders. The presence of grandchildren is often experienced by grandparents as an emotional investment in them by "parent-children" who have left the family home. Infertile children, however, are not able to validate their parents in this way:

I have one brother and one sister. Both have had children. My sister, the eldest in the family, is the mother of four children. My brother is polygamous and is the father of seven children. Each of them has entrusted a child to our parents, who now swear by [my brother and sister]. Praises, blessings, all are addressed to them first and most often by name. Me, they hardly ever mention my name. I benefit only when their prayers are addressed collectively to their offspring. My mother supported me for a few years to help me find cures, but now she doesn't really care. When she sees me, she just says "May God take care of you." (Fanta, Case Study 1)

The fostering of children can benefit elders. Sterile individuals break a chain of vital balance that links them to their parents. Infertility, a form of "symbolic death," disrupts filial ties.

Exclusion from Society

Like Madame HS2, many childless women admit to having felt social marginalization just as keenly as exclusion within the family.

I very seldom go to ceremonies for marriages, and especially baptisms. During baptisms, I feel the full weight of certain people's gazes. Others ask, "When will your turn finally come for us to enjoy such festivities?" And then almost hypocritically, they implore God to dry your tears. (Madame HS2, 31 years old, childless, Yantala district)

Because value systems in Nigerien society are based upon procreation, the fear of being abandoned or repudiated is significant among childless women. This fear is magnified fourfold. Like Muslim Arab women, they face "the dread of empty wombs, terror of miscarriages, obsession with female births, and misfortune of infant mortality," to quote Abdelwahab Bouhdiba (2001: 264). The six women presented in the preceding chapter experienced three of the four fears listed here. Fanta had already experienced divorce and was close to experiencing it again. Lobbo lives under this threat daily. The others could one day make this decision themselves for, as a doctor I interviewed remarked, they are "often backed into their last corner by relatives and other networks of shared acquaintances."

Self-Exclusion

Much more than an individual's relationships to others, infertility affects one's sense of self. Both in the medical environment and in the world of popular and familial care, we have seen that attention is generally focused on the physiological aspects of infertility to the detriment of attending to the psychological consequences. For most patients, this results in intense and lonely suffering, which further heightens feelings of vulnerability.

> I feel like no one cares about me, neither in the family nor elsewhere. I often wonder if certain people don't even hate me. When you're alone, people don't really think about asking after your health, people don't think about checking in with you. Even if no one has ever opened their mouth to push me aside, I've understood it through their behavior. (Madame HS2, 31 years old, childless, Yantala district)

Bodo Ravolomanga reports similar attitudes of marginalization and self-exclusion in Madagascar: "This sidelining can come from herself or from those around her. Feeling uncomfortable in her community, she finds it difficult to make a place for herself that corresponds to her age and her sex" (1992: 77). Infertile women may feel more comfortable being around younger girls and young men and lose touch with the worlds of married women, deepening their distance from them. It is difficult, however, to draw a clear line between what women in despair perceive and the intentions of those around her. Contradictory feelings alternate in the infertile woman.

THE GRIP OF SHAME AND GUILT

To simplify the analysis of what are two related and complex emotions, I could distinguish between the feelings of shame and guilt by considering that in the first case the "social court" faces the individual, while in the second the individual in search of a child prosecutes and judges herself. Guilt here is not a matter of fault but, in the case of the sterile person, of disability—a breach of a social duty. As for shame, I will use this term to refer not to immoral conduct but rather to indicate the notion of "face," as in "losing face," which produces feelings of embarrassment. I focus on concrete situations where one can find values that "approximate" shame (Olivier de Sardan 1984: 35).

Shame and guilt coexist and are complementary; I do not oppose "cultures of shame" against "cultures of guilt." I attempt to be as true as possible to the stories and testimonies of my respondents while respecting their inconsistencies as well as their ambivalences. This approach is inspired by the work of Fatoumata Ouattara (1999), who critiques the way shame is discussed in the literature. Most theorists, whether culturalist, evolutionist, progressive, Judeo-Christian, or ethno-centric, set up a binary between guilt and shame. In her work, Ouattara sets aside oppositions between the "internal" sanction linked to guilt and the "external" sanction of shame in order to trace the broad semiotic field these concepts engage.

The "Debt of Life" That Renders Women "Guilty"

In some women, the inability to give birth and therefore give life induces a strong sense of guilt. This feeling is present in the daily lives of many women without children. From their lamentations and stories, it emerges that they feel that they have failed in a mission—they have not made good on a promise; they have not honored a debt. Psychologist Monique Bydlowski conveys this sense of reproductive debt: "Life is perhaps not a free gift but carries with it the requirement to pass on what has been given. The gift of life, simultaneously a promise of immortality and of death, would imply that a debt is passed from mother to daughter" (1997: 169). An infertile woman thwarts or even annihilates the transmission of this debt. From this cardinal mission that she has not accomplished, and which is perceived as an incapacity, arises an immense feeling of guilt. The idea of unpaid debt emerges in the following interview extract:

> Madame, it's like taking a loan from someone, but afterwards you can't repay it. Whenever you see this person, you feel bad, you feel embarrassed as if you did something wrong (*Baaki jin daadi, jinkin na mutua. Kina ganin kin yi laihi* [H]). This is the case for a woman who hasn't had children. As soon as you're in the presence of others, or even when you're alone you have regrets, you feel at fault. Do you understand what I mean? For each woman, it's a duty to give birth to children. While others fulfill this duty, you sit there watching them. . . . In failing to pay this debt, you feel bad. (Madame FM, 30 years old, childless, teacher, operated on at the Central Maternity Hospital)

In an interview with another respondent, the internal pain that one feels when one is unable to carry out a certain task is stressed:

> For women, motherhood is like a job that you've been asked to do and that you must do. If you don't, you feel indebted. It's a debt you have to pay. If you don't do it, you'll feel wrong deep inside. You consider yourself very wrong because you've thus shown that you're incapable. You didn't respect your duty. (Madame GS, woman pregnant with her second child, Lakouroussou district)

Women seeking to have a child feel anger, denial, guilt, self-pity, resentment, and even jealousy toward those who are already mothers. This psychological disturbance heightens emotions and disagreements with others, making it difficult to live in the same household. Even the most minor problems may take a dramatic turn. We thus return to the susceptibility of the sterile woman mentioned above:

> As soon as the situation of women who don't have children, or women who have many children, or even certain topics related to motherhood are brought up in conversations, I immediately have the feeling they want to humiliate me. I put myself in a sorry state. I shut myself in my room, angry with everyone, for long periods of time. My first seven years [of experiencing infertility] were really painful. Little by little, I found myself with almost no friends. Now I'm beginning to understand that I have to free myself from this weight and think about it less. Because the more I think about it, the more I suffer. (Madame HZ2, 42 years old, childless, Kirkissoye district)

> Now, any encounter with pregnant women tears me apart; it's really painful for me. It feels to me as if they were sent to me by who knows what mysterious force to torture me and remind me that I haven't been able to give birth. The more I see them, the more my belly cries to the child, demands a child. My God! When will I have one? (Lobbo, Case Study 3)

The terms *taali* (Z) and *laihi* (H) used by many of the women I interviewed, such as Madame FM above, express the idea of fault. This is the case for Madame HZ2, who has never conceived:

> You often have the impression that you've done something wrong, you blame yourself, and other people also blame you for not having given birth. (Madame HZ2, 42 years old, childless, Kirkissoye district)

Poor self-perception results from the internalization and acceptance of social norms. The absence of children is accompanied by "an overvaluation of the motherly profession and an affirmation of their vital need to be mothers in 'their flesh and blood.' If, behind this imperative duty we detect the engine of their determination, this duty also gives consistency to an internal tyranny from which they cannot seem to escape" (Santiago-Delefosse 1995: 158).

The infertile woman's feeling of guilt is linked to a feeling of inferiority, of perceiving herself as missing an attribute relative to women-mothers. Lobbo's words "I feel less of a woman" or "I am incapable" express this sentiment of inferiority but also highlight a framework of self-judgment and a refusal to accept oneself. This sense of inferiority then leads to a devaluing of the self, feeding a lack of self-confidence.

An Epistemological Approach to Shame: To "Be Ashamed" Is to "Lose Face"

With the Other's look the "situation" escapes me. To use an everyday expression which better expresses our thought, I *am no longer master of the situation.* (Sartre 1943: 265)

Erving Goffman attempted to draw together the whole fabric of daily relationships by describing and analyzing the units of natural interactions. He presents an interaction as the moment an individual loses autonomy over their representation. Subject to a permanent normative order, the individual's behavior always attempts to adjust to it. Mutual respect for appearances is undoubtedly the most fundamental element of the exchange. Goffman proposes a modernized social psychology in the spirit of Émile Durkheim: "the individual's personality can be seen as one apportionment of the collective *mana*, and . . . the rites performed to representations of the social collectivity will sometimes be performed to the individual himself" (Goffman 1967: 47).

Childless women grapple with their own judgments and those of others. Before letting my respondents express themselves, I analyze the feeling of shame using Goffman's notion of "face." Goffman defines "face" as "the positive social value a person effectively claims for himself by the line others assume he has taken during a particular contact" (1967: 5). He goes on to note, "A person may be said to have, or be in, or maintain face when the line he effectively takes presents an image of him that is internally consistent, that is supported by judgments and evidence conveyed by other participants, and that is confirmed by evidence conveyed through impersonal agencies in the situation" (1967: 6–7). Goffman's concept of "face" enables us to understand how childless women see themselves in light of how they appear to others.

Infertility is a condition that constantly calls into question and upsets the affected individual's subjectivity. This subjectivity is all the more affected when confronted with other subjectivities, whether individual or collective. In social interactions we are constantly in contact with others whose gaze, even when approving, constitutes a kind of prison. Stricken with infertility and feeling guilty for having what is socially deemed a flaw (even if this is neither intended nor premeditated), the infertile individual is always in the grip of feelings of culpability and inferiority. They feel as though they are constantly losing face. Controlling the impressions of others is by no means an easy task, especially since the woman cannot know the place she occupies in the perceptions of the other. This then leads her to oscillate between "cowering and bravado" (Goffman 1963: 18). Eminently social, the feeling of shame is embedded in the individual's daily existence.

"I Feel *Haawi* Because I'm Unable to Have a Child"

In Zarma the term *haawi* is used to convey the feeling of shame. Olivier de Sardan wrote at some length about the multiple meanings of the concept of *haawi*: "Shame (*haawi*) is perhaps the cardinal value of 'nobility' which, symmetrically, negatively defines 'captivity.' Free men have this privilege, slaves are not aware of it. *Haawi* connotes a whole series of meanings, which in French would translate as modesty, embarrassment, decency, good manners, respect, shame" (1984: 35). For him, shame is a central Songhai-Zarma concept:

> "Shame" is central to social behavior; to avoid shame is to be benevolent, modest. . . . Shame thus appears as a safeguard, and this concept crystallizes the strongest social values; cowardice, theft, adultery, and breach of the rules of hospitality or the codes of familial respect all are situations which generate shame. (1982: 183–184)

This concept encompassing reserve and modesty is widely, and perhaps universally, shared in Niger. *Haawi* can be translated as *kunya* in Hausa, *nongu* in Kanouri, *takarikit* in Tamasheq, *pulaaku* in Fulfulfe, and *hayila* or *ebi* in Toubou.

Many interviews show that women who have not given birth have a feeling of *haawi*. This shame is related to the difficulty of keeping face in life's everyday interactions. It is based on an "internalization of behaviors" (Ouattara 1999). The word "shame" is employed in multiple ways, if not excessively, in this interview excerpt:

> I'm overwhelmed with shame when people around me talk about pregnancy, childbirth, caring for children. I've known nothing of all that. Filled with shame, I don't dare speak. I often pretend I'm indifferent so as not to draw attention to myself. Knowing that I'm sterile, it would be sad and shameful if people's talk lingered over me. . . . It's a shame not to have children because then you give

proof of your incompetence to everyone. (Madame HZ2, 42 years old, childless, Kirkissoye district)

To be empty, as some of our interlocutors have claimed, is to lack something, to be incomplete. It is a state of atrophy, which also causes one to lose face. Infertility indeed seems to conform to Goffman's (1963) understanding of stigma. For Goffman, perception and dignity are intimately linked, which is also true for certain respondents:

When you meet some people, they scrutinize you without end, from the bottom up as if you were covered in sores. Many of these people only want to see you with a rounded stomach and nothing else. Without that, you're nothing (*nin wo manti hay kulu* [Z]). (Madame ZI, vegetable seller, 39 years old, childless, Kalley-Est district)

For some of our respondents, shame manifests itself as embarrassment; it pushes one to be reserved, to be discreet, to adopt a low profile in the presence of others, to do everything possible not to draw attention to oneself.

I'm very uncomfortable when people look at me or when they talk about my problem. I prefer to be left alone in my corner to manage my grief. (Madame GD, housewife, 47 years old, childless, Wadata district)

When a woman does not find a positive social role for herself outside of motherhood, how is this feeling of shame managed? According to clinical sociologist Vincent de Gaulejac, who studies the psychology of shame in the life histories of his patients in France, pride is called upon in response to shame:

Pride is the means to restore the Ego, to regain lost dignity, to restore the Ideal self to its pedestal. . . . There is a reversal toward its opposite, an inversion of terms and feelings which transform the internalized negative gaze into an exalted positive consciousness. . . . Pride is an exaggerated narcissism, self-obsession, a reassertion of a self that has been profoundly called into question. (1996: 248–249)

I did find that some childless women seemed to display some pride. Some of them, for example, told me they did not feel like less of a woman than mothers, even though others in their circle contradicted their words, describing their daily distress. Feelings of pride cannot be sustained constantly; its emergence is circumstantial.

LOSS OF SELF-CONFIDENCE AND SELF-ACCEPTANCE

The experience of motherhood enables a woman to become more self-confident, to assert herself in front of her husband's family, to integrate into the group, and to reach a higher status. For a married woman, to share the highly valued identity of a fertile woman, to know she is socially elevated is a necessary attribute for success and self-confidence. Being infertile leads to a loss of self-esteem and respect for one's own personhood. A person feeling thus humiliated may withdraw into a nest of her own creation. The ego gains in confidence under flattering conditions. The infertile woman's ego is pitied and condemned. This is why a devaluation or "pejoration" of the ego—signs of feelings of incompleteness—is common in infertile women. The words of Fanta (Case Study 1) illustrate this decline: "I moved and did things with much less confidence than before. Yes, I was no longer sure of myself." Madame ZI conveys the depth of this loss of confidence:

> I'm no longer at ease, I'm looking for myself all the time. I want to raise my head and be proud of myself among other women. Alas, I can't. No matter how hard I try, nothing helps. (Madame ZI, 33 years old, childless, woman operated on at the Central Maternity Hospital)

Ay si naanay ay bon ga (Z) and *ban yarda da kai na ba* (H) are expressions used to express the lack of confidence common in childless women. The Zarma term *naanay* translates as "confidence." *Ay si naanay ay bon ga* was a leitmotif in the life stories of Madame HS2 and those of her childless peers. "Being proud of yourself," "being sure of yourself," and "having confidence in yourself" all fall within the same register of representations. Because they see themselves as lacking self-confidence, doubt and indecision characterize their behavior. Deeper analysis shows that behind this absence of confidence is a feeling of self-rejection or at least of difficulty in accepting oneself.[3]

TORN BETWEEN HOPE AND DESPAIR

Many sterile or childless women are overwhelmed by multiple contradictory feelings, some of which are hard to pin down. Throughout my

---

3. Editor's note: In Hausa *yarda da kai* means "to have self-confidence" or, more literally, "to approve of oneself." *Ban yarda da kai na ba* is the negative—to reject oneself or lack in confidence.

conversations with them, women navigated between hope driven by an instinct for survival and despair driven by an equally deep sense of defeat. This ongoing tension reflects inconsistent external influences. While some individuals encourage them to fight relentlessly against infertility, others (especially certain healthcare providers) attempt to dissuade them and terminate their quest for treatment.

> I tried everything: marabouts, healers, medicines from great traditional healers, the knowledge of elders, and the medicine of the Whites—but nothing helped. I've told myself it's the will of God, so I might as well resign myself. But it doesn't last long, I just let time pass. I pick up my fight again particularly when I find that my period is about a month late, you see. . . . So I start to hope again, then my period comes, and I get discouraged. It's really difficult to explain, because still other times when my period's late, I tell myself I may be likely to get pregnant and I go back to looking for treatments. But the doctor told me he can't do anything for me because he's already operated on me twice. I try again in other ways, I stop, I start again; it's been going on like this for 16 years. And then there are people who tell me about the miracles of God. They tell me to believe and that it might happen one day. They tell me there are women who have remained 10 years, 15, even 20 years, without children but that one fine day their nightmare came to an end. I also see women around me who tell me they've tried everything without success; when you hear them, you have no desire either to continue treatment or to believe in miracles. . . . What can you do, Madame, when in one ear you hear "there's nothing we can do against fate," and in the other "rise up and God will help you." (Madame MA, 42 years old, patient at the Central Maternity Hospital)

Curiously, among the women surveyed, those who were educated seemed to give in to discouragement more easily after receiving unsuccessful biomedical treatment, including those who had tubal obstructions or who do not ovulate.

> When your tubes are blocked, I don't see the miracle that can make you give birth. I believe in God, but not in such miracles. (Madame NF, social worker, operated on once, 38 years old, childless)

The less scientific a woman's understanding of human reproduction is, however, the more hope she maintains. She seeks treatments with a sense of anticipation, but she is not always optimistic. If a woman believes in fate, she might give up the therapeutic fight, whereas another might not admit defeat because of belief in God or in magic. For the latter, there is no place for paralysis—her handicap is perceived to be a temporary test that she hopes to transcend one day. Thus, Madame RS, who has been married since the age of 16, does not seem overly tired by her long 13-year quest for successful treatment:

> When you have hope, you can always triumph. I think this suffering will one day be a distant memory. God never abandons his creatures, which is why I still believe. I won't stop the treatments. I try everything that family or friends bring me. I ask other women who have also experienced my suffering and whom God has finally helped. I try to follow all the paths they've taken. (Madame RS, 29, woman who came to the National Center for Reproductive Health [Centre National de la Santé de la Reproduction] for a consultation)

While the notions of "capacity" (*hini yan* [Z] and *iya wa* [H]) and "incapacity" (*hina-baano* or *gazante* [Z] and *kasawa* [H]) surface regularly in conversations with both mothers and infertile women, infertile women more commonly employ the words *bon kaano* ("lucky" [Z]) and *bon futo* ("unlucky" [Z]).

CONCLUSION

I have shown in previous chapters how inconsistent social judgments regarding the status of infertile women can be. Often the common notion that infertility is a punishment or a curse can coincide with commiseration, as Laurence Pourchez finds in Creole society, where "sterility is experienced as a tragedy, an ambiguous situation in which the woman is both the victim and the accused; she is pitied, but she is also suspected of having committed—either consciously or not—a forbidden act and therefore of being responsible for her condition" (2002: 71).

Infertile women express a wide range of feelings. Like other physical and psychological disabilities, how infertility is treated is subject to a variety of social customs. The world of "normal people" runs counter to that of "stigmatized people," who are constantly confronted with the gaze and perceptions of others; and this is particularly the case for women who have not given birth. For this group, guilt is also combined with a feeling of incapacity—in spite of their own desires—preventing them from fulfilling the obligations and functions "naturally" assigned to them.

Infertility upsets and destabilizes the status of a woman not only in the home but also in society, generating anxiety. The female body, whose power depends upon bearing children, creates a breach in the transmission of norms, values, practices, and acquired knowledge of all kinds. Psychologically and emotionally, women unconsciously appropriate and internalize a set of beliefs and representations that leave them feeling guilty. Infertility constitutes one of the deepest crises a couple can face. It threatens the relationships of each individual to those around them (relatives, friends, acquaintances, neighbors) and to their dreams for the future. For psychologists or psychoanalysts, infertility causes a "narcissistic wound" that raises the fundamental question of female human identity (Delaisi de Parseval and Janaud 1983).[4]

4. Editor's note: The phrase "narcissistic wound" in this context does not imply a pathological self-absorption but rather an injury to the sense of self that leaves the sufferer feeling exposed and devalued.

PART II

Tensions in the Clinic

CHAPTER 5

Confronting the Biomedical Sphere

Healthcare provision in Africa has been the subject of quite a few con-temporary anthropological studies (Fassin 1992; Gruénais 1996; Hahonou 2000; Gobatto 2001; Olivier de Sardan 2001a; Jaffré and Olivier de Sardan 2003). However, interactions in the context of fertility management are rarely documented. The forbidding intricacies of healthcare bureaucracies are particularly conducive to medical violence. This is especially true in maternal and infant health services clinics (*protection maternelle et infantile* [PMI]) and maternity hospitals, where harsh clinical action and disrespectful language are particularly associated with gynecological examinations and childbirth (Jaffré and Prual 1993; Moussa Abdallah 2002; Moussa 2004a, 2004b; Souley 2003). Yannick Jaffré and Jean-Pierre Olivier de Sardan emphasize that

> In many cases, the violence observed is not separable from the power to treat. Rather, they correspond to "abuses" of this power. Many behaviors of and treatments given by health personnel take the form of outgrowths, more or less illegitimate, of powers inextricably linked to medical knowledge. (2003: 340)

Asymmetrical and hierarchical power relationships profoundly shape the interactions between those seeking healthcare and health professionals (Moussa Abdallah 2002; Moussa 2004a, 2004b).

Employing biomedical approaches for the management of fertility in Niger is generally seen as a last resort. Before seeking clinical treatment, many women have, as they put it, "tried everything" (*ay na ay hina kulu te* [Z] or *na yi iyakan kokari na* [H]) within their family, with traditional

Yearning and Refusal. Hadiza Moussa, Edited by Alice J. Kang and Barbara M. Cooper, Oxford University Press.
© Oxford University Press 2023. DOI: 10.1093/oso/9780197662113.003.0006

healers, or with marabouts. In the realm of infertility treatment, medical practitioners evince very little interest in the three conceptual ways of approaching health issues, namely, disease (the biomedical attestation of the problem), illness (its psychological experience), and sickness (its social significance) (Zempléni 1985). In health centers, the treatment of pathologies takes precedence in the therapeutic relationship. During gyneco-obstetrical consultations, doctors prioritize and often take an exclusive interest in biological pain and symptoms, even as the patients strive to express other complaints. Psycho-social stress and the lived experience of pathology are thus ignored in the management of infertility: steps are taken to treat the disease without really showing an interest in the patient (Jaffré 1997).

Women who seek to regulate their fertility through contraception also face difficulties in dealing with the biomedical sphere. My research shows that the overall biomedical management of fertility remains marginal in Nigerien health centers (Moussa Abdallah 2002). Contraception is inadequately integrated into reproductive health management, which is focused far more upon improving maternal and infant outcomes in childbirth. Tension between clients and staff and the fear of the violation of privacy render the examination table fearsome. Nevertheless, some women do regularly seek out contraception from health centers.

CLINICAL PROCEDURES AND COSTS FOR TREATING INFERTILITY

When doctors consider the social and psychological dimensions of infertility, they do so only marginally. In his critique of the deficiencies of practices in biomedical settings in West Africa, Jaffré insists that "a holistic approach to pathology calls for the consideration of impairments in the body, the physical inability to perform certain tasks, and social handicaps. Faced with serious conditions (sterility, fistulae), one of the caregiver's tasks includes—even if the physical treatment fails—trying to reduce the patient's social disadvantage by addressing the problem as it is experienced" (1997: 17). From my observations, the treatment regimen for managing infertility brushes aside important elements of a woman's condition and does not satisfy what is required of a holistic approach. The fragmented nature of the standard medical approach to infertility is evident from the very first consultation, which covers

1. The patient's reproductive history (e.g., contraceptive practices, pregnancies, births, miscarriages, abortions)

2. Previous medical treatments (e.g., hormonal anti-sterility treatment, surgical procedures)
3. The husband's reproductive history
4. The co-wife's reproductive history, if applicable

In general, the therapeutic relationship is shrouded in ambiguity. During the consultation, the staff make little or no reference to sexually transmitted infections (STIs) when they seek out their patients' histories. Even when sexual habits are mentioned, it is done obliquely, as if the nursing staff find the topic embarrassing. Yet, a patient's sexual history is likely to shed light on the causes of her infertility. If infertility is the result of a venereal disease, which is quite common, the reticence of the caregiver (who leaves such questions out of the interview) and of the patient (who evades them when they are asked) leaves the diagnosis ambiguous. This is also the case with women who, because of their early entry into sexual activity, have used contraception for a long time, which often has real sterilizing effects.[1] Sexuality and infertility are linked, and when the relationships between the two are hidden it can empty the gynecological consultation of any real substance.

Of the various medical treatments, I will discuss tuboplasty as it is the main one offered in Niger. The other available procedures are preliminary diagnostic interventions.

Celioscopy: An exploratory technique in which an endoscope (a tube fitted with an optical system) is introduced through the wall of the abdomen with the intention of observing and taking samples of the abdominal organs.

Hysterography: A procedure for X-raying the uterus following the injection of an opaque substance.

Hysterosalpingography: An X-ray of the uterus and fallopian tubes following the injection of an opaque substance. This radiological examination is a combination of the hysterography (X-ray examination of the uterus) and the salpingography (X-ray examination of the fallopian tubes). This is the most common preliminary

1. Editor's note: HM makes a surprisingly strong claim that long use of contraception can lead to infertility without offering sources or explaining her logic. The train of thought seems to be that women who use contraception are likely to engage in sex with multiple partners, which exposes them to the STIs that can lead to infertility. But the link to STIs here is not the use of contraception; it is having multiple concurrent sexual partners.

procedure done in the first stages of infertility detection and treatment in Niamey's associated care centers. In the Nigerien medical environment, the hysterography and hysterosalpingography are designated indiscriminately by the standard term "*hystéro.*"

Tuboplasty: Prescribed in the treatment of female infertility, consists of clearing blockage from the fallopian tubes, often following an infection. Tuboplasty to clear a blocked fallopian tube is the one procedure that can reverse infertility in the medical arsenal at the Central Maternity Hospital in Niamey. It requires a surgical procedure. Tuboplastic surgeries are the most commonly performed procedures at the Central Maternity Hospital.

Unlike most other medical procedures, cesarean sections and gyneco-obstetric operations were significant sources of revenue for the centers that perform them at the time of my research. Depending on the type of operation, the rates charged at the Central Maternity Hospital (including hospital costs and the purchase of products) ranged from 25,000 CFA francs to 100,000 CFA francs (see Table 5.1). The average base salary for a teacher at that moment rarely exceeded 60,000 CFA francs (91.46 euros).

A system of monthly rebates to health center staff, proportional to the amount brought in, encourages care providers to perform expensive

Table 5.1 PRICING FOR MEDICAL PROCEDURES AT THE CENTRAL MATERNITY HOSPITAL IN 2006

Procedure	Price (CFA francs)
Normal delivery	15,000
Celioscopy	35,000
Cesarean delivery*	35,000
Curettage	10,000
Ultrasound	3,000
Forceps delivery	25,000
Hysterosalpingography (outpatient HSG)	25,000
Tuboplasty	55,000
Sutures	10,000
Hospitalization (category 1)	25,000
Hospitalization (category 2)	15,000
Hospitalization (category 3)	4,500

Note: *The government of Niger decreed that cesarean sections at the Central Maternity Hospital are to be provided free of charge starting in February 2006. Hospitalization costs are measured in five-day renewable packages. *Editor's note*: At the end of 2006, 498 CFA francs was equivalent to one US dollar.
Source: Financial Department of the Central Maternity Hospital, February 2006.

procedures. The rebate is a type of bonus paid by the healthcare establishment to its agents. In Niamey's various care centers, the basis upon which the rebates are calculated is as follows: 40% of revenue is paid to the state, 35% is distributed to agents in the form of rebates, and 25% is kept by the health administration to ensure, among other things, the purchase of cleaning products.

Interviews carried out in Niger's medical environment, and in particular at the Central Maternity Hospital in Niamey, shed harsh light on the commercial character of fertility management in all its aspects (pregnancy, childbirth, infertility treatment). The frequency of performing expensive procedures is an indicator of the high level of commercialization in healthcare. Some women have experienced two, even three successive tuboplasties to no effect. The pressing and obsessive demand for women's maternity is coupled with the highly incentivized position of the medical staff. In the French context Santiago-Delefosse emphasizes that the pressure upon women to make use of in vitro technologies and upon hospitals to perform procedures creates a cycle of emotionally painful repeated attempts (1995: 1–2). However, sometimes in Niger hospital staff impose surgical procedures beyond what women seem to have requested:

> At my first appointment, the doctor said to me: "we might have to operate on you." He prescribed a painful examination with a tube in my genitals.[2] When I returned for the third time, he said: "Prepare yourself ma'am, you'll be hospitalized for the operation." I wasn't very eager to have this operation but ended up accepting. At the end of the day, he never asked my opinion. (Madame AS, 27 years old, childless, Maourey district)

In the hope of a happy outcome, some women accept treatment plans with no knowledge of the real consequences. Fertility management in the medical environment represents a market enterprise that generates resources for healthcare structures and their staff. Many users (patients and those who accompany them), consider certain practices abusive as they often go far beyond the framework of clinical necessity. For this woman undergoing an operation, who spoke to me in French, "There are shortcuts that care providers often take in order to prescribe surgical procedures. They might offer them as early as the first or second appointment" (Madame ZI, 33 years old, childless, woman operated on at the Central Maternity Hospital).

2. This might refer to either a hysterography or a hysterosalpingography.

The hospital staff's lack of openness with me, on the one hand, and the patient's lack of informed judgment (due to ignorance or insufficient understanding), on the other hand, limit my analysis of overtreatment. Nevertheless, in another area of fertility management, that of assisted deliveries, the question of overtreatment arises quite seriously. For example, caregivers may administer oxytocin inappropriately because they can charge for it (Jaffré and Olivier de Sardan 2003). Similarly, cesarean sections, which are recommended by the World Health Organization in maternal and infant health centers to avoid infant and maternal deaths, are often improperly recommended to patients.

The more revenue a health facility makes, the higher the returns for its staff. I estimate the average monthly bonuses received by a non-auxiliary health worker to be around 5,000 CFA francs. Examining the methods of remunerating staff, I have sometimes wondered about the merits of these practices. Many facts support the claim that the incentive system encourages caregivers to take out their scalpels for monetary gain. For example, some women scheduled to undergo a cesarean operation end up giving birth by natural means while the materials for the procedure are being prepared; I have identified up to seven such cases. My observations, as well as patient testimonies, suggest that cesarean sections are more and more motivated by the nursing staff's mercantile interests. Madame Malam HS sees herself as an "escapee of the cesarean section." She recounts the following:

> I had a long labor that lasted more than two hours. One of the *lokotoro* women assured me I could give birth naturally with a little patience. She didn't stay with me because her shift was ending. The new *lokotoro* was a younger man. After reading something in my file, he ordered them to move me to another room. He came to me and said, "Madam, we're going to operate on you. It's the only way, the baby's tired, he can't come out normally." There, I really panicked. A few moments later, when everything seemed ready for my transfer, I pushed hard, in one last burst. The baby almost fell because no one believed a natural birth could happen. Two doctors who were taking care of another woman hurried over to deliver my baby. I had a small tear, but that's better than being cut open. Meanwhile my husband had left to get the money for the operation. (Madame Malam HS)

These types of accounts are common. Convinced that the pursuit of profit drives these types of prescriptions, some think it would be wise to create a framework to protect consumers against abusive practices. This is an idea shared by certain "enlightened" women who have bad memories of their stays in the care centers, the Central Maternity Hospital in particular.

> I think patients who are taken advantage of should create an association to show medical staff that there are limits. They might ask for reparations if, for example, you're given an unnecessary cesarean section or when an operation is done poorly. It's done elsewhere, so why not here? (Madame FM, 30 years old, childless, teacher operated on at the Central Maternity Hospital)

THE DECISION-MAKING PROCESS SURROUNDING CLINICAL PROCEDURES

Female patients, as well as their therapy management groups (which may include a woman's husband and other members of the extended family), often submit to medical authority in the decision-making process surrounding care. Across different maternal and infant healthcare centers, many clinical procedures are in fact carried out without the patient's agreement. They are performed either unilaterally or without the patient's knowledge.

The most crucial decisions, such those regarding a cesarean section, salpingectomy, hysterectomy (following problematic deliveries), and certain surgical interventions related to infertility treatment, are often made *without the prior consent* of the interested parties (patients and their relatives) under the guise of an emergency. This urgency does not always seem to be as real as providers want to make patients believe. The decisions of care providers are prioritized to the detriment of the preferences of those concerned. An emerging theme from my interviews is that "everything is a pretext for an operation." It is no coincidence that surgical operations (cesarean sections in particular) are commonly designated by the evocative term of "sacrifice" (*hiida* [H]).

> *Ay maternite sentral gidan hiida ne* ([H] The Central Maternity Hospital is a place of sacrifice). (Madame IA born BS, 25 years old, giving birth, Gaweye district)

In addition to the material profit mentioned above, the discretionary power of medical personnel sometimes takes precedence over the desires of patients and those around them (husbands, close relatives, etc.). As the following interview excerpt indicates, a woman underwent a hysterectomy without being informed in advance:

It seems that a woman who's had three cesarean sections isn't supposed get pregnant again, but I don't know if they have the right to cut maternity short after a single operation. When my delivery went poorly, the doctor "inverted my uterus" I think.[3] After the procedure, a nurse simply told me: "after the operation they just did, you can no longer have children." Besides, we don't even know who was responsible for this mistake. I remember it was a Chinese man who performed the surgery, but I don't even know his name. His name must be on the papers. . . . Even today, we don't know who it was. They decided I can't have any more children. Do you think that's normal? (Madame FM, 50 years old, housewife, three children, Gaweye district)

When it comes to the medical treatment of infertility, many patients say they do not know how certain treatment protocols work. For example, I have encountered patients who believe that tubal obstructions were falsely diagnosed in order to prescribe costly surgical procedures that then proved unsuccessful. Some who have traveled abroad to continue or resume treatment have been surprised to learn that they have undergone treatments that are inappropriate for their conditions. Madame IS is one of these women:

I was told my tubes were blocked by a fibroid. I had an operation. Usually when the fibroid is removed, it's shown to the patient and the person accompanying her as evidence. I wasn't shown anything, even when I asked. None of the nurses wanted to answer me. Every time, I was referred to someone else who referred me to another person, and so on. I still had no children two years later, so I went back. They told me my tubes were still blocked and that I'd have to have surgery again. I told them I needed time to find the money. We talked about it at home and decided I should go to Côte d'Ivoire. There they said I didn't need an operation because my tubes were clear. And I ovulate normally. . . . They asked my husband to be examined. At first he didn't want to, because he'd just remarried. But when my co-wife still wasn't pregnant after a year, my husband underwent a treatment that was very successful. In Abidjan, they detected that he didn't have enough water.[4] . . . I almost had surgery twice for no reason. They take a lot of money and they don't provide care. Now I have a child and the next one won't be long. (Madame IS, 29 years old, one child, Talladjé district)

3. Hysterectomy, the surgical removal of the uterus, is commonly designated in local languages by the expression "inverting the uterus." Editor's note: The image is of a container that has been turned over so that it can no longer be filled.
4. The patient probably refers to an insufficient secretion of sperm.

Other patients, like Madame IS, told us they had been slated for surgical procedures as early as their first meeting with a specialist. In these instances as well, no transitional treatment was provided before the procedure.

> They did my surgery at the start of my consultations. The doctor said that if I've been childless for five years, it's because my tubes are blocked. He said that without even "looking" at me.[5] I thought he should've done an X-ray. He said it was okay because the machine was broken. And they operated just like that. They said they'd opened the child's path. I've been waiting for a pregnancy for three years. (Madame HH, 37 years old, childless, Collège Mariama district)

In light of these declarations, we can deduce that in maternity hospitals preference is often given to haste and even amateurism in the care of patients and their conditions. According to some patients, the one-sided decisions made by doctors regarding their treatment have done more harm than good.

> I had an operation for a cyst at the Central Maternity Hospital. They left part of a compress in my body. For six weeks, the doctors only prescribed medication to ease the pain. I had to harass them until they agreed to do a more detailed examination. They brought me back into the operating room, where they made an incision to take out the piece of compress. (Madame HS2, 31 years old, childless, Yantala district)

If, in the case of cesarean sections, urgency often influences decisions and thus frees the resulting care procedures from a slow decision-making process that could prove fatal to the mother and/or the child, decisions surrounding other procedures could certainly be made jointly between healthcare personnel and the users (patients and their family circle: spouses, relatives, etc.). Yet, skipping the step of proposing treatment, care providers make the decisions, and patients must agree whether they want to or not. In the vast majority of cases, the only obstacle to treatment is financial. Indeed, some patients refuse or postpone treatments because they cannot afford them (clinical procedures, hospitalization, purchase of medication, etc.).

> I'm sure the doctors are making money from us. Between the appointments, the operation, and prescriptions, I've spent more than 100,000 CFA francs. They barely listen to you but make you spend a lot of money. This means

5. "Look" here corresponds to "consult physically."

they're interested in the money and not the treatment of your problem. (Madame ZI, 33 years old, childless, woman operated on in the Central Maternity Hospital)

Patients are neither provided with sufficient health information nor given the opportunity to make well-informed decisions.

THE LIMITS OF THE MEDICAL MANAGEMENT OF INFERTILITY

I got married when I was 21 and I've been waiting for a child for 11 years. Twenty months into our marriage, my husband married one of his cousins. They had four children. At the end of our first year of marriage, I began to worry and go to the Central Maternity Hospital and to marabouts and healers that my aunts recommended. During all these processes, my husband never helped me. It's often difficult for me to get taxi fare from him. In 2001, I was operated on for a tubal obstruction, which cost me more than 130,000 CFA francs.[6] But my husband didn't give me anything. On his family's side, some do tell me about the go-to people they know about. When they hear of an effective healer or marabout, they give me his address. (Madame MT, art seller, 32 years old, childless, Sonni district)

Just as the entire fertility process is addressed as a matter of interest to the extended family, multiple parties can be called upon in dealing with infertility. From among the families of the two spouses, some people are solicited and mobilized more than others, mainly other women in the woman's family (aunts, sisters, mothers) and, more rarely, women from the husband's family. Men seem uninterested in these initiatives as they seldom provide assistance to their wives. Their involvement in the pursuit of various therapeutic approaches rarely exceeds the allocation of some financial resources to their wife.

My husband often gives me money when the doctor orders many tests. But more often than not, I manage on my own small income. (Madame ZI, vegetable seller, 39 years old, childless, Kalley-Est district)

Men who accompany their wives or support them against all odds to keep them in the household are very rare:

6. Editor's note: About $220 at the time. The per capita gross domestic product in Niger in 2001 was about $820.

and they're often castigated by their relatives. And in many cases, these types of supportive actions don't last long. They're ephemeral, unlike the commitment of a wife, who is often more loyal in supporting her partner through adversity. (Madame ZI, 33 years old, childless, woman operated on at the Central Maternity Hospital)

The indifference on the part of husbands toward their wives' reproductive health is not a figment of the women's imagination. This lack of care is illustrated in cases when a woman develops postpartum genital fistula, a birth-related injury.[7] After the emotional first weeks or months of seeing the complications that fistula causes, many men leave and eventually repudiate their wives:

Men can be assured that wherever they go, they won't lack in offspring. For example, when a woman is ill, her husband rarely assists her for more than three to five years. But when the reverse occurs, a woman may continue caring for her husband for more than 20 years. She won't leave him, either. The man flees immediately when his wife falls ill, forgetting that she contracted this illness while in the marital home. Only her children care for her. Their father will start his life over with another woman. I know so many examples of this. One of my friends had complications during her first delivery; she has urinary incontinence. Only five months later, her husband took a new wife and sent my friend back to the village where she now lives with her parents. This has been going on for three years. (Madame FM, 50 years old, three children, companion of a woman giving birth, Gaweye district)

When no children have been born after a man has remarried once or twice, there are situations where the man takes an active part in the search for infertility treatment. Because male infertility is usually concealed, the men who experience it hide their pursuit of treatment from their close relations. They provide moral and financial support to their wives, while at the same time taking care to keep their own actions from view.

My cousin-in-law SY married two other women in addition to my cousin. None of them gave birth. They quickly left to build their lives elsewhere. My sister, who

7. Editor's note: Women in Niger who develop fistula after prolonged labor also experienced tragic obstetric outcomes (stillborn children or babies dying within two days of delivery) (Meyer et al. 2007). Women with fistula in Niger report being depressed, having suicidal thoughts, and becoming divorced (Alio et al. 2011; Maulet, Keita, and Macq 2013).

loves him very much, stayed with him and it's been nine years. SY understands that the problem comes from him and that it's been the reason for the failure of his two marriages; he helps my sister a lot. She's often the one who secretly brings him back from the treatments he's trying. But during the first four years of their life together, my cousin was left alone to face her grief. The family helped her a little bit financially. Everyone, starting with her, was convinced she was infertile. I think she will eventually leave if they don't find a good solution. She's only 33 years old. She can still have a child. (Madame SM, 26 years old, two children, student, Sonni district)

Men's indifference to their wives' therapeutic pursuits is closely related to the blame placed on women regarding infertility, an imputation which is further reinforced by recourse to polygamy. Regarding the husband's involvement in the process of caring for an infertile wife, my findings are consistent with those of Fatou Sow and Codou Bop:

It is important to underline that the woman takes on every stage of the "obstacle course" that constitutes the search for treatment of infertility or sterility almost entirely alone. Too often, she benefits neither from the physical presence, nor from the moral or material help of her husband, nor from his solidarity. On the contrary, the only solution that he brings to their common problem is polygamy, which he hastens to adopt by marrying one or more women. (2004: 165)

More generally, family assistance is in evidence only in the overall management of *successful* fertility (sexuality, pregnancy, and contraception). This interventionism, however, disappears when it comes to finding an effective treatment for failed fertility. Indeed, the majority of childless women interviewed said their loved ones did not provide them with significant help. Overall, these women think that family networks "speak more than they act":

Family members talk a lot, become very sad as well, but they do very little. (Madame ZI, 33 years old, childless, operated on at the Central Maternity Hospital)

Family guides you and gives you information, and that's all. (Madame IM, 43 years old, childless, Balafon district)

Aside from my mother, who often brings me remedies to try, the rest of my family doesn't contribute anything but psychological support. (Madame FM, 30 years old, childless, teacher, operated on at the Central Maternity Hospital)

Even among family, it's hard to find people dedicated to helping you materially. An aunt or sister can drive you to the doctor or the marabout, but it's you alone who has to "pay up." Yet during baptisms or marriage ceremonies, these same people can ruin themselves for you. If you want the commitment of those around you to be total, become a mother. (Madame RA, companion of Madame FM)

Some respondents perceive the traditional therapists they turn to for dealing with infertility as taking advantage of their predicament. They argue that gullible patients suffering psychologically can be skillfully exploited by marabouts or traditional healers. Jaffré's observations uphold their sense of vulnerability: "Even if it is sometimes possible to consider these contributors as offering symbolic and psychological support, it is unfortunately often demonstrated that these familiar characters from the Sahel benefit from the distress of their clients" (1997: 11). In biomedical settings the suffering of infertile women does not lead to dependable psychological support.

CONTRACEPTION IN THE CLINICAL CONTEXT

So far, we have focused upon the issues of under-fertility and childbirth. In the same way there are tensions between health personnel and patients over infertility treatments and delivery, there are a host of problems that arise when women seek contraception at health clinics.

The contraceptives common in Niamey's health centers include condoms, oral contraceptives (pills), injections, intrauterine devices (IUDs), and implants.[8] The condom became common in Niger with the advent of HIV/AIDS. Condoms are used almost exclusively in non-marital encounters and are easy to buy from street vendors. They are associated more with the fight against sexually transmitted disease than with the prevention of pregnancy. Interviews suggest that neither women nor men like to use condoms because they dull pleasure. Additionally, the use of condoms is associated with sexual debauchery and adultery. During my observation in a health center, when a midwife asked a patient with an unplanned pregnancy, "why wouldn't you use a condom since other methods have failed?" the patient answered, once out of the room,

God forbid it comes to that! We'll never use those plastics [condoms] made for *gabdi* ("seductresses" [Z]). Using those things is like bringing Satan into the

8. The diaphragm is not widely known by respondents or healthcare providers. Spermicides and vaginal suppositories are, like the diaphragm, little known and little used.

family. How dare they propose that to an honest mother? No, we'll never use those plastics. Besides, this kind of thing has never been a topic of conversation between my husband and me. (Madame SH, 36 years old, five children, housewife, Balafon district)

The IUD is very often feared by women and little used in Niger, although it is available. Norplant is the only implant that has been tested at the National Center for Reproductive Health (Centre National de la Santé de la Reproduction [CNSR]) and is not yet widely known outside Niamey. Because it can be detected under the skin, few women want to risk their husband discovering they are using it.

Injectables have the advantage of being discrete. The most common injectable product is Depo-Provera, referred to simply as *cansa* (Z) and *alluura* (H) ("the injection") by most women. Women often prefer injections to oral contraceptives because they are invisible, don't need to be hidden, and limit the need for frequent visits to health centers.

My husband doesn't know that I'm taking contraceptives. Once every three months, I go to the PMI in secret to have my injection. With the pill, you often have to go every month. (Madame DA, housewife, Niamey)

Of all the available contraceptives, the most commonly used one is the pill, referred to as *kini* ("tablet") in Zarma. Apart from literate patients who cite specific varieties of pills, for example, Lo-femenal, Minidril, and Stédiril, most women make little distinction between the different categories of pills. Some differentiate the pill prescribed for breastfeeding women from that taken by women who are not lactating.

At the time of my interviews in Niamey, the price of a pack of pills for a complete cycle varied between 300 CFA francs at a health center and 1,000 CFA francs at a pharmacy. Women living in peri-urban areas can obtain them on the street for 100 CFA francs.[9] In either case, prices are "reasonable," and sometimes women who reject contraception on the grounds of expense contradict themselves in admitting this:

Spending 300 or 1,000 CFA per month to guard against an unwanted pregnancy, that's not bad. (Madame FK, 31 years old, woman giving birth, Maternité Gaweye)

9. Editor's note: In 2005, 300 CFA would have been worth roughly 60 cents.

For many of my interlocutors—health workers and users of contraceptive products—the sums required are manageable and modest in light of the preventive utility of contraception. When first legalized, contraception was free as part of an effort of intensive popularization of new methods of birth control. The first public family planning programs benefited from the financial and logistical support of international organizations (such as United Nations Population Fund, US Agency for International Development, and United Nations Children's Fund) that provided early users with free access to contraceptives. Today's contraceptives are only expensive relative to the free contraception distributed in the past (Moussa 2004b).

OBJECTIONS TO BIOMEDICAL CONTRACEPTION

Rumors about medical contraceptives prevent women from making use of them. Although the accepted rationale behind both popular and medicalized contraceptive practices is ensuring the physical well-being of a woman and her children, many women fear that certain types of contraception (particularly medical contraception) will affect their bodies negatively. The fact that today pharmaceutical contraceptives can be acquired from street peddlers has contributed to the spread of rumors. Observing these dynamics in Nigeria, Koster explains that women are hesitant to use the pill, IUDs, and Depo injections because they are given little counseling on their effects or how to use them from peddlers or medical staff: "Contradictory stories circulate about their adverse side effects, ineffectiveness, and impairment of future fertility" (2003: 302).

Women who have the courage to break religious and social taboos to use contraception face dissuasive voices. Healthcare personnel, either for lack of time or inadequate discussion, do not clearly explain the side effects. The adverse side effects women report experiencing may be due not to the contraception itself but to drug interactions. The pill is feared by potential clients for various reasons: risks of inter-menstrual bleeding, obesity, heart attack, hypertension, cancer, or the formation of fibroids (and therefore secondary infertility). This interviewee, for example, believes the growth of uterine fibroids to be linked with taking the pill:

> Today, people are talking more and more about fibroids. Many women have operations for this problem. There's an explanation. These women usually take the pill. These drugs, as you take them, pile up at the bottom of your stomach, more specifically in the uterus. In the long run, this is what keeps these women

from having children. (Madame FK, 31 years old, woman giving birth, Maternité Gaweye)

The rumors about injections and oral contraceptives are more or less the same, but the probability of a woman remaining permanently infertile is much more commonly associated with injections.

> I was told that injections can be dangerous because a woman who uses them can become infertile. I've even heard they use it in some countries to sterilize women. (Madame HD, 27 years old, married, two children, seller of telephone cards, Talladjé district)

The use of the IUD is most often associated with infections of the reproductive system or unwarranted inter-menstrual bleeding. If there is bleeding, women may believe that it is because the small copper device is dangerous. Another notion about the IUD is that it "migrates" inside a woman's body to end up in the stomach or other locations of the body. These concerns, some of which are reasonable, could be addressed through better communication between patients and caregivers. In particular, the importance of good hygiene to prevent infection does not appear to be explained sufficiently to patients.

INHOSPITABLE CLINICS

The chilly reception clients receive in clinical settings is at the heart of difficult patient–caregiver relationships. Almost no inquiry on the health system can escape this concern (Jaffré and Olivier de Sardan 2003; Konan et al. 2005). Whether in the context of pregnancy and birth, the treatment of infertility, or the pursuit of contraception, personnel minimize or ignore the quality of patient reception, while patients emphasize it as a problem. The level of hospitality does not seem to patients to meet even minimal expectations of social communication:

> Midwives treat us with little consideration. First, when you enter a room, they usually just gesture to the table where you'll be examined. It's like you don't deserve to be spoken to. They speak in a tone like you'd use when addressing your children (*I ga salan ni mata kan ni bunbo donu ga salan ni izey se* [Z]). There's no respect in their conduct. You could count the polite ones on one hand. (Madame HD, 36 years old, two children, member of a singing troop, Talladjé district)

At family planning consultations, the atmosphere is always tense. In the year that I've been coming to this PMI, only once has a caregiver smiled at me and taken my child's hands. It was also the only time I really felt comfortable. She spoke to me as if we'd known each other for a long time. I didn't feel intimidated like I had every other time. But I never saw that woman again. Maybe she was new. In general, they're not very warm (*i si ga walwala* [Z]). Even if they aren't openly arguing with you, they aren't welcoming either. (Madame SM, 30 years old, five children, housewife, Boukoki district)

Jacques Cosnier proposes an interactionist approach to care relationships that is inspired by the work of Erving Goffman. A medical consultation should begin with an "opening" (including greetings and the offer to sit down), and it should end with the "closure" (taking of leave and ending the consultation) (Cosnier 1993: 22). His model offers a protocol for the treatment of patients:

Opening
Definition of the problem (asking of questions)
Examination
Diagnosis
Discussion of the diagnosis
Additional tests/examination
Prescription
Closure

Comparing this schema with observed interactions within health centers, I noticed considerable divergence from the ideal. My prolonged presence in health centers while conducting multiple studies (Moussa Abdallah 2002; Moussa 2004a, 2004b; Souley 2003) has made me aware of the gap between the ideal and the actual practices and habits among caregivers, producing a local professional culture that resembles what Olivier de Sardan refers to as a "privatized bureaucratic culture" (2001b). In conversations with patients, complaints about the quality of their reception are very frequent.

You're tense, you never know what might happen. The midwife is usually on edge. You only see her smile when she receives someone she knows or someone as important as her. (Madame HI, 23 years old, housewife from Téra, evacuated to the Central Maternity Hospital)

Women who are marginalized by such poor reception experience it as a form of devaluation: *kaynandi/kanya yan* (literally, "humiliation, shrinking"

[Z], from *kayna*, or "small"). Hausa-speaking women also refer to *wulakanci* ("humiliation").

> Going to consultations at a medical center requires a prior understanding of how the system works. For those of us in the countryside, we experience an extreme devaluation (*iri ga di ka kayna yan* [Z]). If they know you are from the country-side, they don't even deign to show you around the center to tell you where the showers are, for example. You have to run into a compassionate Muslim if you want any chance of orienting yourself in a health facility. But when they realize you're just as good as they are—that they're no better than you—they treat you well. The preferential treatment people from the city receive is because they have education. If you're educated, you think it's a waste of time to talk to people who don't know anything. When you're educated, you know everything. That's not the case for an illiterate person who has a hard time telling their right hand from their left—especially if they aren't fluent in Hausa and Zarma. Even a little bit of education, through primary school, means you will be well looked after. Also, if your pockets are full, people will take care of you. Illiterate people are unfortunate. (Madame FM, 50 years old, three children, companion of a woman giving birth, Gaweye district)

Patients often experience this lack of empathy among caregivers as a betrayal of feminine solidarity in the face of shared conjugal and social constraints to fertility management.

> We're all women, and for that they surely understand the challenges we experience within and outside our homes. Some women come in secret, without their husband's knowledge. For this, they need support from the midwives. Others, like my case today, have serious problems with their cycle. They need a minimum of understanding from midwives. Instead, most of them behave as if they're not also women who give birth, have children, and space their own births apart. Yet the trials of women are all shared (*ay ciiwon mace duk daya ne* [H]). (Madame FO, 28 years old, three children, housewife, Ouallam)

By contrast, with members of their own family, allies, and acquaintances, caregivers certainly do know how to exhibit kindness (Moussa 2004a: 51). Jaffré characterizes midwives using the metaphor of the chameleon "tuning their behavior to a particular environment without consciously thinking about it" (2003b: 305). As Michèle Lacoste writes, "depending on the type of hospital, the service, the doctor, and according to the degree of familiarity, authority prevails over courtesy, and distance prevails over proximity" (1993: 48).

Poor Communication

During contraception consultations, when information is conveyed to patients it may be too vague, or there may be none at all. The hurried pace of consultations gives little time for communication (Moussa Abdallah 2002; Moussa 2004a, 2004b). Many patients say they are hungry for more information and health education. Immediately after an introduction to the different methods available in the center, for example, the patient is presented a pack of white pills and told they must be taken every day. Then the healthcare provider tells the patient, "when you've finished taking these white tablets and as soon as you start on the brown ones, try to come back here for your next dose." The caregiver insists particularly and only on the regularity of the dosage: "Don't forget to take one tablet every day, and I mean only one." As for injections, nothing specific is explained to patients apart from communicating the three-month period of effectiveness. They are simply asked to come back if by chance they notice an abnormality in their menstrual cycle, for example, the occurrence of inter-menstrual bleeding.

Regarding the IUD, patients are usually asked to come back for a checkup that takes place two or three months after the first placement, with no guidance on hygiene beyond the remark that "the rubber [IUD] is not for dirty people! Above all, you must be careful to be clean."[10] This exhortation to cleanliness could, for the less educated patient, refer to washing regularly, wearing clean clothes, or having a tidy and clean house. A nurse trainee at the Gaweye Maternity Hospital, aware of the inadequacy of the communication, remarked,

> When we vaguely ask women to be clean, they try to do so, especially when they come to the health center. They'll take a shower and dress well before coming here. They take much more care of their physical and external appearance, I really mean external . . . and often—excuse me—well . . . between their legs, it's a disaster. Sometimes even their underwear is disgusting, let alone the rest. There are still many women who don't look after their personal hygiene. It's a question that deserves more awareness. But what do you want? It's not always easy to take time for it. (Madame AI, nursing intern)

10. Editor's note: The French term for the IUD is generally *le stérilet*, but in common usage the hormonal IUD may be referred to as a "rubber" because it is made of a flexible plastic. The expression has no relationship to the English slang word "rubber" meaning "condom."

Both because the nursing staff want to save time and, perhaps, to avoid moments of embarrassment, they prefer to skip the details of cleaning oneself. For midwives, more than other aspects of the family planning consultation, translating how to maintain personal hygiene into words is uncomfortable:

> You can ask a woman about the date of her last period. And as for monitoring her contraception, we can take the liberty of asking her if she might've had sexual intercourse on the day she was probably ovulating. But it's much more difficult for me if I have to give all the details of cleaning yourself. (A midwife, CNSR)

The absence of real communication means that consultations are generic. Yet different patients do not all have the same sexual and reproductive histories. The information given to an educated woman should differ from that given to another who cannot read or write. As this instructor of a training school for health professionals states,

> Nursing staff lack adequate training in adult education to transmit health information to illiterate patients who are not, for example, able to use medical documentation and materials (leaflets or memory aids).

Dwelling on the transmission of this kind of information might make it possible for the midwife to help patients develop practical strategies to remember to take a pill every day. One educated patient felt this type of approach could be easily integrated into a care plan:

> It's very difficult for many women to take the pill. Personally, I think they should have thought of teaching its users little tricks to help them remember to take it every day. Health centers should have communication committees that think about these things. (Madame SA, postal agent, Plateau district)

Unbearably Long Waits

At different health centers and for a multitude of reasons patients feel they are wasting their time. An important element of seeking care is how long the visit will take, given that women spend a great deal of time in health centers seeking treatment for ill children, vaccinating them, getting pre- and post-natal checkups, giving birth, seeking contraception or infertility treatment, and managing their own illnesses. According to patients, the factors that lengthen waiting include, among other things, the late arrival of midwives at care sites, transportation issues, the method of selecting patients, and disregard for the order of appointments (Moussa Abdallah 2002). Health providers sometimes give the impression of spending more time on their cell phones than on their responsibilities. Lengthy breaks for meals are also a source of friction:

> They seem to leave their homes hungry. They take a long time to eat. When they get together to eat their food, there's no way they are thinking about their patients. Meanwhile, we wait, and our housework awaits us too. And too bad for the person who dares to complain about it because then she can forget having a consultation. If the midwife refuses to see you, who can force her to? I think no one! (Madame OH, 34 years old, six children, housewife, Gaweye district)

Visits by friends take precedence over patients at times. Women particularly resent the failure to respect the order of patients by arrival time. It is experienced as a form of injustice, as the words of this woman suggest:

> The midwife can call in someone who arrived long after you. That woman might be admitted as an emergency simply because she knows someone in the hospital: the midwife, the nurse, or even the guard. While you're waiting quietly with a number, someone who's just arrived from home goes before you, without a number. That's not right. We all put our activities on hold to come to the health center. Our concern is to leave as soon as possible. . . . It's as if we've come just for the walk. (Madame AG, 43 years old, braider, Kollo)

Concerns About Modesty and Violations of Confidentiality

Above all, women fear the betrayal of their privacy or *haawi* (propriety, modesty, decency) (Ouattara 1999). Any violation of *haawi*, often linked to the inappropriate gaze or proximity of others, gives rise to feelings of shame and unworthiness. Patients believe that midwives should respect their sense of modesty and privacy.

> A *lokotoro* who has *haawi* respects your feeling of *haawi* when it comes to talking about your intimate problems. And to show that she has *haawi*, she must make sure that the conversation you have during a consultation remains between the two of you—no one other than she should hear what you entrust to her (*ni asiro kan ni go feeri a se* [Z]). (Madame AG, 43 years old, braider, Kollo)

Whether during childbirth or during family planning consultations, patients feel that the minimum conditions of discretion are often not met in care centers.

> For *lokotoros* it's as if it's normal, completely natural to speak publicly about your sex life or to expose your body to the eyes of others. Even if you can tell it to a caregiver, that doesn't mean it should be known by everyone. (Madame OH, 34 years old, six children, housewife, Gaweye district)

This violation of modesty can also have a psychological impact on patients. This is especially the case for patients who come to a first family planning consultation and are asked to undergo a gynecological examination. This was the experience of one woman from a small village:

> The first time I came, I was asked to undress and I was ashamed. I removed my camisole and my *pagne* but kept my underwear on. The *lokotoro* told me to take it off. I couldn't do it, so she sent me away. (Madame GS, 24 years old, from Day Kaina, Tillabéri)

Even for women who are accustomed to health centers, gynecological exams are not always easy when the caregiver is accompanied by other colleagues:

> I had an IUD and was in a lot of pain. So I came back to the Central Maternity Hospital to check what was wrong. The midwife asked me to lift my *pagne* in front of four people: one of her colleagues, two room attendants, and a person I couldn't identify because she didn't have a smock. The five women were chatting in front of the consultation bed. The bed wasn't even surrounded by its fabric [screen]. When I got on the bed, they were still there. I was reluctant to lift my skirt because I was hoping they'd leave. But no, apart from one room attendant who left hurriedly—I think someone called her—all the others stood there staring at me. That was when I told the midwife that I didn't intend to strip in front of an audience (*ay si hini ga fata koonu jama jine* [Z]). She just said to me, "either you want me to look at your problem, or you make your own rules and I won't." Without another word, I took my file and left. I never went back there for the same problem because I had the IUD removed at [another] center. (Madame OH, 34 years old, six children, housewife, Gaweye district)

Some of the most shocking betrayals are in the realm of privacy. According to one patient (LM), her husband found out she had been taking medical contraception because a midwife had not exercised restraint and had disclosed information concerning her among acquaintances.

Many patients have a very negative perception of nursing personnel. But how do caregivers regard their patients and those who seek contraceptives? Do patients comply with even the minimal requirements given by healthcare workers? Are patients as blameless as they consider themselves to be?

"BAD PATIENTS" AND THE TRANSGRESSION OF MEDICAL STANDARDS

Some patients at maternity hospitals and PMI centers—whether intentionally or not—provoke confrontations with nursing personnel. The category of "bad patient" is a construction on the part of caregivers to characterize three types of behavior: provocation, non-compliance with instructions, and irregular attendance to appointments.

Because of the widely shared negative stereotypes of nursing staff, some patients come to consultations "conditioned in advance" to behave aggressively (Moussa Abdallah 2002: 69). As one midwife saw it,

No one ever thinks a patient or client in a health center is at fault. A few months ago, I asked a young woman being treated for post-abortion hemorrhage to be calm and hold still [*se tenir tranquille*] for her tests so as not to risk hurting her.[11] I had to perform a curettage. All it took was for her to hear the word "calm" [*tranquille*] for her to get angry. She said, "You mean to imply that I'm not calm, that I've prostituted myself and that I'm getting rid of my child. Well guess what? I'm married." She went into an indescribable rage. She took me to task in a matter of minutes. It's true that some of our colleagues have made inappropriate comments about patients during childbirth. But from there, to generalize these behaviors to the whole medical world doesn't make sense. Many people refer to past experiences and come here with preconceived ideas. We midwives are seen as the embodiment of the devil. I find this to be neither fair nor true. (A senior technician in obstetric care, Central Maternity Hospital)

11. Editor's note: In West African French, particularly when referring to children and women, the command to *se tenir tranquille* carries the sense of being well behaved. A *fille tranquille* is a "nice girl," whereas a woman who is not *tranquille* may be thought of as loose, restless, a party girl.

In another account, a caregiver recalls advising a 46-year-old woman who had just had a miscarriage to start using contraception to protect her own health:

> [T]his lady read into it too much; she immediately upbraided me for trying to lecture her. She made a direct link with her sexual activity, which she thought I was trying to judge. But I wasn't even thinking about that, and it's none of my business. All I know is that pregnancies like hers cause many problems for both caregivers and patients . . . . It is not uncommon for *grand multipara* women to die in childbirth, and that's in addition to the various other ailments they experience.[12] . . . I had to defend myself and I didn't give in. I made it clear to her that I was doing my job and that another caregiver would have told her the same thing. (A midwife, Gaweye Maternity Hospital)

Most conflicts occur between healthcare workers and patients of less privileged backgrounds. In the context of family planning, however, patients from the middle classes and occasionally those from the upper classes can be "difficult." Healthcare professionals find these more privileged women to be "the most combative."

> I remember when a teacher—I don't know if she taught middle or high school— berated one of our nursing colleagues who had criticized her for coming five days before the expiration of her quarterly [contraceptive] injection.[13] . . . She told our colleague that she could even teach her a thing or two, that she wouldn't be intimidated like the others. By that, she meant the poor patients. (A nurse, CSI, Boukoki)

Some patients who come for family planning consultations do not observe the recommended dosages, whether out of negligence, omission, or, as sociologist and doctor Isabelle Gobatto puts it, their lack of "receptiveness to medical rationality" (2001: 152). This raises the problem of the ignorance of or the transgression of biomedical paradigms (Gobatto

---

12. Editor's note: *Grand multipara* is a technical term referring, generally, to a woman who has had seven births at term or close to term (more than 20 weeks' gestation). There is a great deal of debate on the subject, but they are generally seen to be at greater risk of maternal and neonatal complications (malpresentation, placenta previa, low or high birthweights, postpartum hemorrhage, perinatal death).

13. Editor's note: It is not clear what "expiration" refers to precisely. The shots should be administered every 12–13 weeks. It's possible the patient was correct that it was a suitable and convenient time to get the injection, given that the window is roughly a week.

1999, 2001). Women often become pregnant because they did not follow the directions given to them on how to take the pill. One day I witnessed a minor altercation between a patient and a room attendant at the Boukoki Maternity Hospital. The patient said that she found herself pregnant "while taking contraception." The midwife being busy in a delivery room, she explained to the attendant that she had always followed the directions given to her and that she was disappointed to have become unexpectedly pregnant. When I later interviewed her, it emerged that she often took three pills at a time because she had forgotten to take them the previous two days.

> The main thing is to take the number of tablets prescribed. In any case, I always managed to finish the 21 white tablets before my next period. But this time, there was no period. I'm pregnant and my child is still very young. Those ladies don't explain to people well enough. I really wonder if their products work.

This patient did admit that, according to the caregiver's instructions, the tablets should be taken daily. She also recognized that she should only take one tablet per day.

> You have to take one pill each day, but it's also normal to take two tomorrow because you forgot to take one today. And in this case, I don't think that goes against the *lokotoro*'s instructions. Besides, many of my friends do the same thing. I asked advice from one of my neighbors who also told me that this is normal. I don't see the problem. These midwives, *wallahi*, they just don't want to admit they're wrong, that's all. (Madame AH, 27 years old, three children, housewife, Boukoki district)

Women sometimes fail to take the pills as directed on days when they are not having sexual intercourse, thinking there is no point.

> When you and your husband haven't "seen" each other [had sex], I don't see the point in taking the pill. For example, when my husband travels a bit, I don't take the pill. I take a day or two off, for a week or two until he comes back. (Madame ZM, 29 years old, four children, housewife, Collège Mariama district)

A prominent domain in which patients are considered irresponsible is, of course, that of keeping their appointments. Generally, caregivers schedule appointments every 90 days for injectable contraceptives and give a delay of approximately one month (between 27 and 28 days) for oral contraceptives when they do not dispense doses by trimester. Whichever option is chosen, some patients come long after the date of their appointment. Issues of timing are common sources of friction:

> A local woman came to pick up her pills the same day she was likely to be ovulating. She lives next door, hardly 500 meters from here. I suggested that she come back at the time of her period, because I'd understood that she wanted to take them the same day she showed up. Technically that's not how it works. But she became frustrated. And this woman is educated. One of my colleagues who had prescribed the products to her before had taken care to write the date of her appointment in her notebook. I just told her that she should have come on that date. Unfortunately, she had understood things differently or she had done it on purpose—I don't know. She immediately blew up on me and on a room attendant who had the misfortune to try to calm her down. She called us malicious. I say "we" because she was talking about all caregivers. It was silly—we could have reached an understanding, but she had her strong ideas and it was difficult for me to reason with her. She left very angry and never came back.

I also observed conflicts surrounding the placement of or follow-up on IUDs. One woman almost created a serious crisis in a care center following an infection caused by her IUD. She should have come in for a checkup five weeks earlier but had not done so. She likely would not have gone back to the center at all if not for her infection, probably caused by poor hygienic conditions. She complained that the insertion had been done incorrectly. According to the midwife, this infection could have been avoided if she had kept her appointment.

> She came five weeks after her appointment. What's more, she had no concept of hygiene. If she'd come for the checkup, we would have realized that something was wrong and we would have removed it—with her the IUD does not work. That's what we ended up doing. We sent her to the CNSR. Some patients knowingly don't show up for the appointments that have been set for them. We really have become—oh, what's the word—scapegoats. That's it—scapegoats for the whole medical system, because whatever we do, people only see a negative. There's no shortage of bad apples in any profession, but you shouldn't generalize. (A midwife, Talladjé district)

Caregiver–patient interactions give rise, on both sides, to efforts at self-justification and exoneration. Abuses of the relationship are in evidence on each side: just as a caregiver can be perceived as impolite and domineering, there are also clients who staff view as "bad patients." Within the biomedical sphere these two main actors rub shoulders, confront one another, and trade accusations. The behavior of each suggests that there is a "reciprocity of perspectives."[14] If nothing else, it is clear that within the very facilities that should provide women with the best prospects for managing their fertility, there are systemic problems that make it difficult for women to take advantage of the services that are available.

14. Editor's note: HM seems to be referring to the approach of sociologist Georges Gurvitch in using the expression "reciprocity of perspective." See Coenen-Huther (1989) for his place in the field.

PART III

Knowing and Negotiating Contraception

CHAPTER 6

Contraception Outside of the Clinic

The desire to control fertility outcomes, whether for reducing or increasing the number of births, is universal. Despite their wide availability in the capital of Niamey, biomedical contraceptives are in fact little requested or used.[1] In general, contraceptive practices draw on traditional and magico-religious techniques.

In this chapter, I inspect the social norms of birth control and the motivations of individuals who, despite pro-natal sentiments in Niger, seek contraception. Much of this takes place outside of the clinical setting. In Niger, particularly in large urban centers such as Niamey, there are many forms of practical knowledge, each offering a variety of contraceptive methods. I describe the different kinds of natural, traditional, and magico-religious contraceptive methods used in the city of Niamey and its surroundings. Some are passed down through the family as grandmother recipes. As in the reproductive process as a whole, different specialists are called upon in contraceptive practice. I label these non-biomedical contraceptive practices as "traditional" or popular techniques, which themselves can adapt and change.

---

1. Editor's note: In 2022 Avenir Health's Track 20 Project projections estimate that 10.5% of women make use of a "modern" biomedical contraceptive method in Niger (FP2030 2022).

Yearning and Refusal. Hadiza Moussa, Edited by Alice J. Kang and Barbara M. Cooper, Oxford University Press.
© Oxford University Press 2023. DOI: 10.1093/oso/9780197662113.003.0007

SOCIAL NORMS CONCERNING CONTRACEPTION

One cannot understand the usage of birth control without paying attention to the social environment. Doing so allows us to highlight the ambiguities and contradictions that are present in society and affect individuals' lives. In interviews relating to contraception my respondents were often ambivalent, their ideas about contraception unpredictable and ambiguous. The critical importance of fertility gives rise to considerable friction over contraception. While some say they are in favor of contraception for the purpose of spacing births, others reject it vehemently. Regardless of whether an interlocutor regards deliberate birth spacing favorably, open support for limiting the overall number of births is rare. Nevertheless, the traditional and popular contraceptive methods that I will later present give evidence—beyond what people say—of women's (sometime hidden) desire to regulate their fertility.

Choosing contraception involves the consideration of a multitude of factors—the state of one's body, sociocultural expectations, and economic priorities. Some urban families refer to the cost of educating children as the fundamental factor that favored the use of contraceptives. Concerns about the health of the woman and the child can promote contraceptive uptake, but these same worries can also constitute a major obstacle. I examine the logics and motivations that guide and justify the use of any given contraceptive method.

Economic Motivations for Using Contraception

Previous demographic and socio-anthropological studies highlight the economic interest that many African societies derive in producing numerous descendants (Caldwell 1982; Locoh 1984). The economic difficulties faced by many urban families, however, may discourage them from hoping to have many children. It seems that Malthusian thinking may gradually gain ground in a society known for its pro-natalism. The choice, however, to control the number of births is not necessarily at odds with an individual's aspiration to have a sizeable number of children, nor does it imply the rejection of childbearing altogether. Some respondents emphasized economic difficulties—the cost of feeding, clothing, caring for, and educating many children—that were a burden and source of anxiety for couples. As one man put it,

Everything is too expensive in town. And you can't choose to live there and then let your children wander the streets. They have to be educated. If they go to school, they must be fed, dressed, and provided for adequately so they aren't marginalized and they work well. Can you imagine having close to 10 children? Just finding housing would be a real problem if you don't own property! (SA, 36 years old, three children, police officer in Niamey)

For this reason, the belief that "God nourishes every mouth created" bandied about in some religious circles may be eroding. The fear of facing a difficult tomorrow confronts everyone, including both the woman who chooses to use contraception without informing her husband and the one who embraces "natural" reproduction. Yet economic rationales for family planning were almost exclusively invoked by literate respondents from the middle and upper classes. By contrast, people from the poorest classes thought of contraception as a "luxury" that only the educated and wealthy can afford. In truth, economics alone cannot fully explain who adopts contraceptive practices and why.

Birth Spacing for the Wellness of the Woman and the Child

A multitude of terms and expressions convey the long-standing understanding of the need to use contraception to guarantee the health of the mother and her child. This understanding generates support for the spacing of births. As 41-year-old ZG (seven children, seamstress, Boukoki district) told me,

> A mother and her child should be allowed enough time for their bodies to become strong. The mother must recover from the nine months of pregnancy and also from the efforts of raising her child before considering another pregnancy. As for the baby, he must be strong before he has a little brother. Spacing births is in the interest of both.

Common words and expressions that reflect the social norm of birth spacing include the following:

• *fulanzama* (Z) or *huutu* (H). This term signifies the period of rest that a woman must take between two births. Perceived socially as any other job, childbirth and the raising of children require a pause to allow the human body to recover.

- *jandi dan yan hayyan da care gama ra* (Z). Literally, "interval between births" or "spacing of births." This formula may be joined with the term *fulanzama* to convey the need for an interval between conceiving for the regeneration of the female body.
- *nya nda nga izo gaham baano* (Z) or *lahiyar uwa da dan ta* (H). The health of the mother and her child; this phrase captures the sense that the well-being of the woman and her child are conjoined.
- *zanka ma nga nya wa han ga kungu* (Z). The child shall get enough nourishment from the mother's milk. The phrase emphasizes the importance of a woman succeeding in feeding her children enough without the encroachment of a new pregnancy.
- *zankey I ma du ga hini care/zanka ma hini nga kayne sanbu* (Z) or *yara su imma juuna* (H). These expressions capture the sense that well-spaced children can support each other. The priority is that the older children be physically able to carry their little brothers. An older brother should, for example, be able to take care of his younger brother if a "reasonable" time, two years or more, has passed between their births.

The first three expressions—*fulanzama, jandi dan yan hayyan da care gama ra*, and *nya nda nga izo gaham baano*—are today part of a shared discourse used by both staff and clients in health centers. In fact, these terms were standardized to help popularize the usage of biomedical contraceptive methods.

Bad Milk

According to many of my interlocutors, infants, because of the fragility of their young bodies, need sufficient time nursing (two years minimum) to develop before the mother gives birth again. In popular discourse, but also sometimes that of healthcare providers, the unweaned baby of a pregnant woman is at great risk of feeding on "bad milk" (Moussa Abdallah 2002; Moussa 2004b). What exactly is this "bad milk" that does not nourish but rather kills?

A woman who becomes pregnant before weaning a nursing child has *nasu/nasu yan* (Z) or *rurutsa* (H), a pregnancy before weaning her baby (Bernard and White-Kaba 1994: 237). If she has pregnancies close together, she will be called *woyboro kan ga nasu* ("a woman committing *nasu*" [Z]) or *mace mai rurutsa* ("a woman committing *rurutsa*" [H]). The milk produced by a woman who is guilty of *nasu* is referred to locally as "bad milk" because of its purported harm to the nursing child. It is designated by the expression *nasu wa* ("the milk of *nasu*" [Z]) and *nonon kane* ("the little brother's milk" [H]). In Zarma, the term *nasiize* ("the child of *nasu*") is commonly used to refer to the child who drank "bad milk." The baby is a "child who is breastfed while the mother is pregnant again" (Bernard and White-Kaba 1994: 237). In Hausa, one might say of such a child, *da ya sha nono* ("the child drank the milk").

In rural areas, many people consider this milk to be the main cause of infant mortality. Failure to use contraception during breastfeeding, combined with the return to menstruation, exposes women to pregnancy and, consequently, exposes their children to the risk of consuming bad milk. This idea is invoked to encourage breastfeeding women to avoid pregnancy. If a woman becomes pregnant despite these warnings, those around her will recommend that she stop breastfeeding. They must seek out either milk powder or animal milk from goats, sheep, or cows to feed the newly weaned child.

The following mocking proverb is often addressed to women with closely grouped pregnancies: *Ize wo a ma nga nya wa naanu a ga bisa a ma hincin waa naanu* ("It is better for a child to drink his mother's milk than that of a goat" [Z]). Another common expression is *nasiize nya a man hari hay* (Z), which translates to "the mother of *nasiize* hasn't given birth to anything." A *nasiize* is expected to have a limited life expectancy. They are destined die at any moment; therefore, the mother should not count them among her offspring.

Despite the popular expectation that mothers wean such children quickly, I encountered some women who hesitated to wean their children out of shame and for fear of the ridicule of their friends, neighbors, and co-wives. To eliminate suspicions of pregnancy, they continue breastfeeding, temporarily forestalling the shameful revelation of the new condition.

> Many women try to hide the beginning of pregnancy by continuing to breastfeed their baby. The ridicule addressed to *nasiize nya* [a woman who commits *nasu* or the mother of the *nasiize* (Z)] is unbearable. During the first few months, they can divert people's attention. But it's only a temporary solution. (Madame LB, seller of medicinal drinks, Niamey)

In some societies, it is a taboo for a mother to have sexual relations while breastfeeding. Pregnancy in a lactating woman reveals the violation of the social norm of sexual abstinence during breastfeeding. Among Fulani and Gourmantche families in Niger, to respect this taboo, a woman who has given birth is required to remain abstinent for two years in separate lodging from her spouse. Medical anthropologist Sylvie Fainzang observes this expectation of marital abstention from sex among African immigrant women in France: "a woman must not have sexual intercourse while breastfeeding her child because it is supposed that a pregnancy occurring during the period of breastfeeding would stop milk secretion to the detriment of the first child" (1991: 93).

In my conversations, women emphasized that a mother who is frequently giving birth endangers not only the health of her child but also her own health if she does not give herself time to recover. To her various household tasks are added the physiological and emotional demands of her child. Women thereby become less productive, which is crucial to the development of the family (but also of society) in an agricultural or pastoral economy. The challenge of managing the burden of many young children is therefore a deterrent to conjugal sex and to pregnancy for many women. These prohibitions fall particularly hard upon women, as this comment reveals:

> There is often little respect for a woman who is both breastfeeding and pregnant. Both she and her child are strained; the baby through the "bad milk" he suckles, and the mother through the combination of pregnancy and breastfeeding. In this situation, either you feel very sorry for her, or you are dismissive of her. It also proves that her husband's always between her legs. You know what I mean? (Madame MN, 54 years old, seller of aphrodisiac products, Talladjé district)

These standards provide a fairly effective safeguard against closely grouped births, reinforced through proverbs, sayings, and various other formulae that I will explore next.

Popular Depictions of Closely Spaced Pregnancies

There is a strong stigma attached to having multiple births in quick succession. Just as we celebrate the glory of the fertile woman, we castigate the woman who does not space her births and has many children that look about the same age. Building on a previous study of stigmatizing terms and phrases surrounding closely spaced pregnancies (Moussa 2004b), I present here common expressions that draw analogies between women and animals and phrases that comment on women's sexual activity, the health of the family line, and women's appearance.

Women who fail to space well are likened to mice, grasshoppers, and goats—animals known for their prolific breeding:

- *woyboro kan ga hay danga can* and *can ize boobu koy* (Z). "A woman who gives birth like a mouse" and "the mouse with many offspring." Among the mouse species, the black mouse is reputed to be the most prolific as it would seem to give birth weekly.
- *a hay da do bi* (Z). "She gives birth like a black grasshopper."
- *gurma hincin ize* (Z). "The goat of the Gourmantché." The Gourmantché raise a breed of small, prolific goats. Like the mouse or the grasshopper, these goats give birth at close intervals and almost always to twins.

Women who are unsuccessful at moderating their pregnancies hear dehumanizing insults:

> They tell you: "poor goat, you give birth like a black mouse" (*can bi*) . . . or they say, "you're like a *gurma hincin ize*." And it's usually your co-wives or sisters-in-law who throw these proverbs at you. You know, the black mouse gives birth every week. (Madame FM, 50 years old, three children, companion of a woman giving birth, Gaweye district)

The depiction of the overly sexually active woman appears in popular maxims that call implicitly or explicitly for contraceptive use. Through proverbs and metaphors, the woman is challenged to examine her sexual life.

- *Da kamba* (or *kambe*) *mana mooru gorey do kajiyan, kulu kanba ga kande saajora* (Z). Literally, "If the hand is close to the buttocks because it itches, it's obvious that it will touch excrement" (Moussa 2004b: 9). Through this proverb, the *nasiize nya* is reproached for having an intense sexual life prompting close pregnancies.
- *A ba alborey ga daaru* (Z). Literally, "She loves men excessively." A woman who gives in to sexual prompts from her husband or who excites his sexual appetite is considered to be driven by an unbridled sexuality.

We see here how women's fertility, when it is very active and abundant, can incite disgust. In their history of abortion in France, Jean-Yves Le Naour and Catherine Valenti underscore the contradiction that exists between the dominant pro-natalist discourse and the reality that "in everyday life, large families are the subject of, if not contempt, then of reservations with a glimmer of an underlying imputation of bestiality—uncontrolled fertility thus gives evidence of pathological behavior" (2003: 92). In Niamey, men may be criticized by those close to them: "a man whose wife becomes pregnant frequently is often told to go easy" (Madame FM, 50 years old, three children, companion of a woman giving birth, Gaweye district).

Infant mortality is associated in popular thinking with close pregnancies. When a woman falls pregnant while nursing, both the fetus and the nursling are at risk. Through unrestrained sexuality and fertility, a woman threatens the success of the lineage, given the frailty of the children produced:

- *Tagi wi ga zaraw windi/tagi wi ga gine zuure dey, dumi hanna ma koma ni se I laala mo ni si duwa* (Z). This colorful agricultural image means "destroying as much good growth [of millet] as bad growth," calling to mind the farmer whose plow turns over young millet plants instead of weeds.
- *Banda si te, jine si te* (Z). "It doesn't work at the front or the rear." This expression conveys the idea of stagnation in the family's perpetuation. Close pregnancies ultimately destroy all of a woman's children, jeopardizing the prospects for the continuation not only of the household but also of the kin group.

For women there is also a concern for the toll childbearing takes on their bodies, affecting their attractiveness in a context in which the security of marriage is uncertain. This is captured in vivid expressions describing the appearance of the mother of *nasiize*:

- *Zanka go ni se ca bon, zanka go ni banda ra, zanka go ni fuma cire* (Z). This expression literally means "you have a child on your legs, a child on your back, a child under your navel" (in your belly). In Hausa, *mace da goyo da ciki* corresponds to this Zarma expression. Literally, it means "a pregnant woman carrying (a child) on her back," in other words a woman who is both breastfeeding and pregnant. The *nasiize nya* gives the impression that her whole body is covered with small children.
- *Da jiiri kulu bora ga hay bora ga te zara-zara no* (Z). "You'll end up like a rag if you give birth every year." This phrase conveys the expectation that a woman's body will degenerate following repeated and close pregnancies.
- *Kazama danga nasiize nya* (Z). "Dirty like the mother of a *nasiize*." The presence of many young children does not allow a woman to maintain proper hygiene (of her body, her clothes, or the home).

This disdain for the female body overtaken with childbirth corresponds to a sense of a pathological lack of control by the women themselves.

- *Ba alboro na nga mudun feeni a bon, a ga te gunde* (Z). This is said of the woman who has close pregnancies: "she becomes pregnant even when her husband shakes his pants over her."

Helène Deutsch studied the psychological problems of French women patients in the 1940s (when contraception was illegal) who felt that they conceived too easily and against their will. They complained that if a man just looked at or touched them, they would fall pregnant. Such women experienced their immoderate prolificacy as a pathology:

> The biological ideal can paradoxically become an anomaly. This is the reality for women whose fertility defies all efforts made to curb it, and who are pushed to their physiological limits by the challenge of constant reproduction. All their emotional capacity is mobilized in the fight against their fertility, just as the emotional preoccupation of a sterile woman is centered on her inability to conceive. ([1949] 1987: 106)

CONTRACEPTIVE KNOWLEDGE AND PRACTICES AMONG INFORMAL NETWORKS

Niamey's "traditional" networks offer a great deal of wisdom and numerous practices in the field of contraception. To practice traditional forms of contraception requires skills (*dabari* [Z] and *dubaara* [H]) and knowledge that belongs to older individuals, who themselves have learned them from their own kin. But first, I will discuss the natural contraceptive practices that are commonly used in Niger.

Natural Practices

Many practices designed to control fertility seem to be universal (Guillaume 2009; Koster 2003; Andro 2001; McLaren 1990; Flandrin 1984; Gélis 1984; Devereux 1955). I have identified breastfeeding, postpartum abstinence, withdrawal, the calendar method, and post-coital baths as broadly known natural methods of contraception mentioned by my respondents.

The secretion of prolactin, a hormone produced by milk, generally blocks ovulation in breastfeeding women for at least the first six months after childbirth. Women are aware that when they nurse frequently and have abundant milk, their menstruation stops, providing a form of contraception (Moussa Abdallah 2002; Moussa 2004b). Some couples rely solely on the lactational amenorrhea method and do not take additional measures to prevent an unplanned pregnancy. However, this physiological transformation involving prolactin does not occur in all lactating women.

Postpartum conjugal abstinence is a more certain, but more difficult, method to avoid falling pregnant. This consists of "pausing" the regular practice of sexual relations between spouses for a time. Before the advent of Islam, the duration of this suspension could be as long as two years while the baby nursed. With Islamization, the period declined to 40 days, corresponding to the period of the new mother's confinement. While in confinement, the new mother is too "dirty" to take care of certain activities, such as preparing food. Until she has performed the proper ritual ablutions, she is unable to observe certain religious obligations (prayer, fasting, or pilgrimage). It is believed that the blood of new mothers has a corruptive power. The lifting of her confinement at the end of the 40 days marks a transition toward purification. Alms are given, and this event marks the woman's return to sexuality and normal life.

Because of the importance of sexual abstinence and the "impurity" of the new mother, often an old woman from the family's entourage lives with the couple until the end of the confinement. This old woman, commonly called *uwan mai biki* (H) or *antugay nya* (Z), which means "mother of the newborn," takes on a multitude of tasks. Above all, she ensures that the woman who has just given birth strictly observes the rules and prohibitions associated with this period of seclusion, during which she is considered "impure." This "mother of the newborn," who is rarely the biological mother of the woman who has given birth, prepares the water needed to wash the baby and his mother. She manages the feeding of the newborn and that of the new mother quite closely. She may, for example, force the latter to drink large quantities of a beverage intended to fatten her (*hangandi* "beverage" [Z]; *shan kiba* "plumping beverage" [H]). This fattening is intended to produce abundant milk and prolong the period of amenorrhea.[2] In the past, many Hausa women returned to their own mother's home for the period of nursing and sexual abstinence to protect them from sexual temptations.

Many couples, however, do not pay much attention to this prohibition on conjugal sex, especially when the new mother does not have a scrupulous and authoritarian *antugay nya* to enforce it. Moreover, and more commonly, the *antugay nya* might be sent home after the baby's naming ceremony (the seventh day after birth), to safeguard marital intimacy or to

2. Across Niger and particularly in Zarma-Songhay society postpartum weight gain among married women is highly valorized. Generous amounts of millet porridge, and in some cases millet bran, enriched with milk, are provided for the mother. I would estimate that she might drink three liters of porridge per day. Young women compete in stoutness in *hangandi* ceremonies organized after the harvest. Married women who are recognized as "fat" enhance their husbands' prestige.

avoid the expense of offering her obligatory gifts. Some women confessed that they resumed their prayers the day after the child's naming day rather than waiting for the end of the 40-day confinement. The resumption of prayers signals to the husband that his wife is ritually pure and can resume sexual relations.

Many women cited withdrawal, or coitus interruptus, as a contraceptive method. The withdrawal method may be the oldest contraceptive technique in the world, and its use likely transcends culture and religion. In Muslim contexts, withdrawal is known as *azal*, inspired by Arab tradition. In some Muslim settings, the acceptance of withdrawal in Islam has served by analogy as a justification for the use of contraception more broadly.[3]

The calendar method consists of identifying the ovulation period and refraining from sex in that time frame. Calendar methods are mainly used by couples with a certain level of education: those who have attended secondary school (junior high or high school) or higher. Even though there are many ways to calculate that window, the women I spoke with only mentioned one, which appears to be the Ogino-Knaus method, according to which ovulation occurs on the fourteenth day of the menstrual cycle as there is a fertile period from the tenth to the sixteenth day. Many of the non-formally educated women who I interviewed knew of this method but did not explicitly talk about the day of ovulation. Many of them believe that about 10 days after the end of menstruation, the couple should avoid sex for three days to one week. Women who have tried it said that they have been wrong in their calculations and found this method unreliable. This is why it is often used in combination with another contraceptive method. In clinics, patients confess that their spouses rarely adhere to the calendar method.

Another practice that we could add to the list of natural contraceptive methods is washing the vagina with plenty of (preferably) warm water to prevent the progression of sperm toward the uterus. This method, however, is reputed to be the least effective of the natural contraceptive methods.

Family Recipes

One means of preventing pregnancy comes in the form of "family" recipes. The *koira zeeno cambu* ([Z] "pieces of a jug from an old village") was the main

---

3. Editor's note: Despite the awareness of this practice in Islamized circles in Niger, many Muslims (including religious specialists) object to it with the Prophet's assertion that "every soul that should exist on the day of the resurrection must be able to exist."

family recipe cited by women coming from the Zarma villages surrounding Niamey, such as Kollo, Say, Namaro, and Karma. This method was not cited by Hausa-speaking respondents. The *koira zeeno cambu* method resonates with the symbolism of the jug or the gourd, vessels that are strongly associated with the image a woman. Breaking one or the other amounts to "breaking" a woman's fertility. The specialist collects shards from a broken jug found at an old residential site. The shards are used to prepare a contraceptive mixture by pounding them into a powder that is subsequently diluted in a small amount of water. This process is purported to lengthen the intervals between the births of those who consume it. The period of effectiveness for this method depends upon the number of broken pieces: for example, for two years of spacing, it takes two shards; for five years of spacing, five are needed; and so on.

The jug shards can also be brought to a marabout, who "works" them (*a gi goy*), then gives them to the woman, who must keep them under her pillow for the entire duration of her "reproductive pause" (Moussa 2004b). The marabout recites verses or other incantations and performs certain sacrifices. By extrapolation, one healer (AH) explained that to maliciously hinder a woman's fertility, "those who resort to occult sterilizing practices . . . rely heavily on the jug and the gourd."

Self-Medication and Do-It-Yourself Methods

The methods I describe here are carried out by the individual and are essentially forms of self-medication. They aim at the "solitary" manipulation of the rules. To prevent or reverse conception, the woman's objective here is to "make her period come back." Whether the substances used are traditional or biomedical the focus is upon the manipulation of menstruation or "bringing the blood back." As in medieval Europe, the whole enterprise consists of "making blood" (Bologne 1988: 52). All the manipulations are intended to generate menstrual blood, not provoke abortion (Le Naour and Valenti 2003; Gélis 1984; Renne 1997; Koster 2003; Guillaume 2009). Many of my interviewees, however, made little distinction between abortive products and contraceptive substances; the two were almost always conflated.

Within the city of Niamey, the majority of substances used in do-it-yourself methods are derived from plants. Women's exchange of recipes within their networks of sociability and kinship reinforces, as Angus McLaren notes for the case of Europe, "a feeling of female solidarity" (1990: 23). The different substances discussed below often taste very bitter or are very bracing. It is, it seems, the acidity that gives them their contraceptive property.

A commonly used substance is neem leaf. To produce their contraceptive effect, neem leaves are steeped in water, preferably hot, for two to three hours. The drink so produced is to be consumed by a woman after each sexual encounter. In order to increase the acidity and concentration of the product, some prefer to pound the leaves. It is its very bitter taste that gives this drink its birth control properties.

Otherwise, drinking a salt solution after each act of intercourse is believed to have preventative qualities. Additionally, as Pourchez found (2002), women often employ ginger as an abortive and contraceptive substance. It is thoroughly ground and then macerated in water. As a contraceptive, the ginger solution is consumed by the woman before or after intercourse. Taking henna diluted in water after sexual intercourse is also claimed to protect a woman from possible pregnancy (see also Renne 1997). In popular discourse, such methods are attributed the same properties as medical spermicides. Unlike spermicides, they are all intended for women.

CONTRACEPTION PROVIDED BY POPULAR THERAPEUTIC SPECIALISTS

In the popular sphere, marabouts, traditional healers, and itinerant pharmacists supply contraceptive products. Marabouts and traditional healers have certain techniques in common. This is particularly the case with the making of a "contraceptive belt" that women must wear around the hips for the period they do not want to become pregnant. When prepared by either healers or marabouts, the incantation of sacred words determines the duration of contraception. The words *gurumu* (Z) and *damara* (H) generally refer to belts worn for protection against harmful forces. These can be depositories of powerful supernatural forces (Bernard and White-Kaba 1994: 135). Some people also employ the more general terms for a protective charm, *tirayze* (Z) or *laaya* (H), when referring to the belts.

Marabouts produce other types of *tirayze* that may be worn inside the hair or in the bra. Women who do not wear a bra pin the amulet inside the sleeve of their undershirt. This amulet contains scriptures (fragments of the Qur'an or an Islamic text) copied by the marabout. Increasingly, and as a result of what one might call "professional syncretism," one can find traditional healers who also deliver amulets that contain plant substances, often varied, upon which they recite magic words.

Besides amulets, marabouts also prepare *hantum hari* (literally, "written water" [Z]) and *rubutu* or *ruwan allo* ("writing" or "*allo* water" [H]) for their customers. These are verses from the Qur'an transcribed on wooden slates. Once the writings have dried, the ink is rinsed off the slates. The collected inky water is called *hantum hari*. The patients consume this holy water to protect themselves from unwanted pregnancy. In addition to providing holy water, a marabout can perform what is called *addu'a* ("invocation" [H]) and *tufa* (literally, "spit" [Z]). The spittle that accompanies the magic words spoken by the marabout is itself powerful.

The rare method involving both husband and wife requires the sacrifice of a rooster. After having been "worked" upon by a marabout or a healer, the rooster is eaten by both spouses. The "worked rooster" method, according to some of my interviewees, has fallen into disuse as husbands are often uncooperative. As we have seen in fertility management in general, husbands are unwilling to participate in some therapies.

The *Hawari* Technique

The preparation of *hawari* (Z) or *darmu/kulli* (H) involves the making of a variety of ties and knots. More literally, the *hawari* is a "bundle of linen" (Bernard and White-Kaba 1994: 149). Its fabrication resembles other maraboutic recipes (Qur'anic writings in the form of oval amulets) or traditional recipes (bark, herbs, and various other substances crushed and kneaded into balls).

Amulets or crushed substances are placed at regular intervals along a long, wide strip of hide. The strip is closed and sewn so that knots are made in each place where a magical charm is placed. The result is a somewhat wavy belt worn around the hips. Analogous to the ties made on the belt, the womb is also "tied."

Given the prevailing social norms and family values, one might think that this myriad of contraceptive techniques is designed only for married women and therefore only applies to them. There are, of course, discrepancies between prescribed standards and actual practices. Some of these contraceptive techniques, notably contraceptive belts and amulets, are intended for unmarried girls.

The tie or *hawari* comes in two main forms. One can have the power to prevent any sexual encounter from happening in the first place. The second does not obstruct intercourse but prevents pregnancy. To "protect the family honor," parents may ask specialists (marabouts or traditional healers) to carry out the ritual for young girls. This technique consists of "tying up" the girl's stomach, as well as, in a way, her reproductive organs. She is thus preserved not only from undesired defloration but also from pre-marital pregnancy. The following respondent gives some details on the *hawari*:

> There are two kinds of *hawari*. One is against attempted sexual relations outside marriage, and the other is for contraception. If the *hawari* is lost, the girl will never give birth. That's why you want witnesses. When it's not undone, no children. (Madame AG, 43 years old, hairdresser, Kollo)

In Zarma country the *hawari* technique is called *hantiize*. Only *sorko* sorcerors know how to make them.[4]

Often, a young woman wears this belt around her hips without much awareness of its specific purpose, aside from its generally protective qualities. To ensure the wearing of the belt, women are told that it protects against evil spirits, wizards, and other harmful forces. More rarely the secret might be shared between a girl and her mother, and she may be aware that the belt renders her "belly" temporarily unfit for procreation. Even more powerful charms purportedly exist that can be efficacious without requiring the girl to wear them or even to be aware that they exist. Such ties are kept by the parents who commissioned them, and the healer retains a duplicate.

Such belts are to be worn or held in secret until the girl's marriage approaches, when the parents seek out the specialist to neutralize the *hawari*. Its destruction is carried out during a ritual ceremony. In all cases, the specialist (marabout or healer) who initiated the *hawari*, or a person delegated by them for this purpose, must destroy the remnants of the contraceptive treatment; otherwise, the new bride might remain permanently infertile:

> I knew a girl whose parents did *hawari*. I know because the marabout-healer who did it was my brother-in-law. The girl got married three years after he had died, and her mother could not find the duplicate of the cord entrusted to her. Today, she has been married for 16 years and hasn't given birth yet. The co-wife who

---

4. The *sorko* are commonly fishermen. However, for Olivier de Sardan (1982: 341), the semantic field that covers *sorko* is much wider. When we talk about *sorko*, it can be a simple fisherman, "either occasional or professional, or even the 'master fishermen', whose knowledge is inherited from father to son." Some of these "master fishermen" have a magic power which allows them to intervene in dances of possession. It should be noted, however, that not all master fishermen are necessarily fishermen by trade.

came after her is already the mother of five children. (MN, 54 years old, seller of aphrodisiac products, Talladjé district)

If the woman's parents have moved or died without undoing the charms previously solicited, a married daughter may remain permanently child-less.[5] In rare cases, the *hawari* is performed upon the initiative of a partner (fiancé or boyfriend) and without the parents' knowledge. It also seems there are more and more young girls who act on their self-protective reflexes by turning to *hawari* on their own.

The *hawari* intended for young girls can have another use. According to informants, it is possible to suspend the development of a young girl's pregnancy if it has progressed less than three months. Once the girl becomes part of a marital home, the illegitimate pregnancy may be resumed. The main objective is to save the family's reputation by avoiding an extra-marital birth (a tangible sign of the girl's deviation from social norms), guaranteeing that the child will be a legitimate heir.

There are two types of *hawari* intended for married women: contraceptive *hawari* and anti-adultery *hawari*. One interviewee extols the virtues of contraceptive *hawari*:

> Despite the growing popularity of medical contraception, some people continue to use *hawari*. You wear it when you don't want a child; you get rid of it when you want one again. There are also *hawari* that have a limited lifespan beyond which they are no longer effective. Once expired, whether you dispose of it or not, you can get pregnant. Medical contraceptives have their downsides: abnormal bleeding, cramping. All of this discourages some from using them. (Madame AG, 43 years old, braider, Kollo)

The *hawari* technique is also practiced to prevent married women from committing adultery. Appropriate arrangements are made either by the woman, by her husband, or by members of the family:

> There are families that don't just settle for *fatiha* during religious ceremonies where a daughter is married. There are of course things you have to do be-fore; otherwise, it won't work. For example, you can tie it. . . . A girl is tied up

---

5. In these cases, the attitude of the victims varies between resignation and an ex-treme fighting spirit. In the West African sub-region, there are specialists known for their ability to destroy or deactivate such lasting effects. In these cases, women have been able to neutralize their *hawari* thanks to a famous practitioner from Benin or Nigeria.

to prevent a man other than her husband from tempting her once married. Intimacy should be limited to her husband. She must not have sexual relations outside her home. You know with this remedy, even when there's a man who wants to sleep with her, he won't be able to because he'll instantly become impotent. We can find this kind of protection from both marabouts and traditional healers. For us, the Zarma, this is also a form of *hawari*. (Madame FK, 31 years old, woman giving birth, PMI Gaweye)

Referring to the "myth of the sleeping child," women whose husbands are absent for long periods may be accused of using the *hawari* technique to "suspend" a pregnancy that she contracted. Whether in a conjugal or an extra-marital context, through various manipulations of the same sort as *hawari*, a pregnancy might be delayed or suspended, or "put to sleep" just as it can be "woken up" and continue its development. (It should be noted that knots can also be employed to maliciously suspend a married woman's pregnancy.)

Finally, some respondents reported that men, especially marabouts and healers, use the same methods to resist their sexual impulses in the presence of other men's wives. Today, in cities and villages alike, women are increasingly seeking out the help of magico-religious specialists. These specialists often say they are forced to restrain themselves from temptation. These men impose self-discipline through magical processes, allowing them to "put their sexuality to sleep," to protect themselves from desire. The use of this type of *hawari* is effectively an anaphrodisiac.

Many women come here for consultations. They are looking for solutions to their problems. Not just anyone can control himself under these conditions. The temptation is there, present; it is constant. Some of my clients go so far as to try to arouse me. God prohibited fornication. For us, the best way to protect ourselves is to "tie" ourselves. (Alpha O, 50 years old, marabout-healer, Gaweye district)

In general, the use of the *hawari* technique seems to be more widespread in rural areas than in cities. Few hold these secrets as time passes in urban centers. Those who continue to use *hawari* still have strong ties with the ideas and practices of village life. In Niamey, the proliferation of all kinds of charlatans undermines confidence in popular therapeutic specialists (marabouts and healers). If the *hawari* technique seems to be losing steam, it is because, according to one healer, the specialists died without transmitting their knowledge.

Like marabouts, traditional healers craft the *hawari* according to their practice. Their powers derive from such skills as spirit mediation, fishing, blacksmithing, barbering, or hunting. Like marabouts they use incantations (*tufa*). The rituals are often accompanied by sacrifices of milk, cola, sugar, or animals (chickens and small ruminants) at sites such as termite mounds, forges, or the Niger River.

The contraceptive remedies of traditional healers are largely herbal. The pharmacopeia is broadly designated by the term *tuuri safari* (literally, "drugs from trees or plants" [Z]) or *icce* ("tree" [H]). Such medicines may be burned and the smoke inhaled, many are ingested, and the powders can also be enclosed in charms for the cords women wear around the hips or on other parts of the body. Powder from crushed herbs, seeds, or bark may be mixed with milk, water, or porridge.

Substances may also be brewed as a tea before drinking. For example, the milk of a sheep that gives birth to a male lamb at the first gestation may be collected by healers who prepare it with four different plants. After it is made, the decoction is consumed by both the husband and wife. This, then, requires cooperation between the man and woman, as with the worked rooster method.

CIRCUMVENTING THE CLINIC: THE ITINERANT SALE OF MEDICINE

The itinerant sale of pharmaceutical products has expanded rapidly in developing countries, apparently as a response to economic crisis (Chilliot 2003). Didier Fassin (1992) has shown that in Dakar the increase in healthcare costs and the symbolic importance of drugs serve the interests of multinational pharmaceutical companies more than the consumer. Yannick Jaffré (1999) also emphasizes that socioeconomic issues drive the phenomenon of ambulatory pharmacies in Mali. "Street pharmacies" or "ambulatory pharmacies" have become part of everyday life in Niger since 1990 or so.[6]

The sale of these drugs is mostly itinerant. In some cases, it takes place on the edges of public spaces such as markets, bars, bus stations, and health centers. Unlike conventional pharmacies where the customers come to them, it is the salespeople who go to meet the customers, putting time

6. Editor's note: Generally, a young man wanders the main thoroughfares, his pyramid of more or less plausibly packaged biomedicines on a platter on his head.

and effort into entering social spaces (Moussa Abdallah 2001, 2002). They pass in front of concessions, entering compounds, workplaces, or any other areas frequently visited or patronized by potential customers. This informal consumer-directed, door-to-door trade bears little in common with the official healthcare structures with their overly complex procedures for obtaining prescription drugs.

In this context, customers have a better cultural understanding of the itinerant sale of pharmaceutical products (Jaffré 1999). The close interaction between buyer and seller on the street or in the home is more culturally suitable to the context of health. This commerce has its own unique dynamics created by the street pharmacists' invention of an entire language for talking about illness. This lexicon is contextual, inspired, and very convincing. This language shapes and is shaped by interactions with clients around contraception. This "medication of cultural proximity" is often people's first recourse for a variety of ailments (Jaffré 1999: 69). The itinerant pharmacy offers less costly and less complex options to customers who generally come from the poorest strata: they are referred to as pharmacies of the poor with good reason. In their quest to treat general ailments and use contraceptives, people take advantage of the itinerant vendor's physical and cultural closeness (Moussa Abdallah 2001).

In Niamey, itinerant pharmacists sell some contraceptives that are also distributed in hospitals, clinics, or pharmacies (Moussa Abdallah 2001), including the following:

- Condoms: Known as *fuula* (H and Z), or "a man's hat," condoms are the highest-selling contraceptive sold by door-to-door salespeople.
- Oral contraceptives: Known generically as *kini* (Z) or *pilil* (H) (from French *pilule* or "pill," those available are typically Lo-femenal, Eugynon (norgestrel), Ovrette (norgestrel), Stédiril, and Minidril.[7]
- Spermicidal creams but not spermicidal gels or foams.

In marketing these products, peddlers take some liberties. For example, spermicides are intentionally marketed as aphrodisiacs in order to attract buyers. They are thus referred to as *kilen mota da na gida* ("the key to the

7. Editor's note: Oral contraception comes in more or less two forms. Some, like Stediril and Minidril, combine the hormones estrogen and progestin—these are the most effective at preventing pregnancy. However, because the dosage can enter a nursing woman's milk, they are not suitable for women who are breastfeeding. Some low-dose pills are based on progestins and contain little or no estrogen. These are suitable for nursing women—this would be the case for Lo-femenal (norgestrel and ethinyl estradiol), Eugynon (norgestrel), and Ovrette (norgestrel).

car and the house" [H])—that is, the man will be so stimulated that he will want to satisfy every request of his partner (spouse or lover), from handing over the keys to the car and the house to sponsoring a trip to Mecca (Moussa 2004b: 35–36). To offer another example, a contraceptive product sold to women is referred to as the *démarreur* ("car ignition" or "starter" in French). This product purportedly contains elements that can get the sexual machinery up and running. It is also advertised to women as an aphrodisiac. Street vendors woo customers with the product's imagined double benefit as both a contraceptive and an aphrodisiac.

Itinerant pharmacists create close and trusting relationships with their customers, unlike the relationships formed inside health centers. Furthermore, a woman who heads to a maternity center when she is not pregnant immediately signals to all her intention to get contraception. Those who want to keep their contraceptive use out of view of neighbors or close family prefer to use these peddlers, who sell a great many things other than contraception. Safe from judgment, married women, single women, and girls enjoy greater discretion.

Some customers are aware that using contraceptive products from street vendors can expose them to risk through insufficient information:

> When we buy pills from street vendors, the sellers are usually the ones who give us the instructions. Some women ask their friends or acquaintances who have experience taking them. Also, if you've been to the health center once for the same thing, you refer to the dosage you were given at that time. (Madame AH, housewife, Talladjé district)

While the itinerant pharmacy provides customers with the advantages of discretion, affordability, and cultural legibility, there are some significant dangers to its use. Counterfeit drugs abound in this market, as do expired drugs. The spread of inaccurate information about drugs is also particularly problematic.

CHAPTER 7

Negotiating Biomedical Contraception

Control over human reproduction, that is, sexuality, pregnancy, child-birth, abortion, and contraception, entails complex social processes. The planning of births through biomedical contraception—the focus of this chapter—generates conflict and requires negotiation. Contraceptive use goes beyond the microsocial framework of the individual, the couple, or the family and extends to the macrosocial level of the state, conservative religious movements, and public health structures. In the city of Niamey, biomedical contraception is often framed as a new "Western" model that competes with the old methods of fertility management. Opposition to biomedical (as well as other kinds of) contraception often arises out of a fear that the continuity of the family line will be broken.

Despite spousal, family, and conservative religious organizations' opposition to the use of medicalized forms of contraception, women find ways to take up biomedical contraceptive medicines. Women are not passive and resigned victims. The microstrategies that women employ to use biomedical contraception form the primary subject of this chapter. But first I will outline the national political debates surrounding family planning through medicines such as the pill. In comparing normative discussions about sexuality and what happens in reality, a significant gap between ideals and actual sexual behaviors emerges.

Yearning and Refusal. Hadiza Moussa, Edited by Alice J. Kang and Barbara M. Cooper, Oxford University Press.
© Oxford University Press 2023. DOI: 10.1093/oso/9780197662113.003.0008

POWER STRUGGLES AND DEBATES OVER BIOMEDICAL
CONTRACEPTION IN NIGER

The development and spread of biomedical contraception are part of a global movement for social change. The advent of medical contraceptive methods has given rise to new images and symbols relating to sexuality, reproduction, and social relations between men and women (Moussa Abdallah 2002: 100). This "contraceptive revolution," in its medicalized form, is often perceived to be imported (Andro 2001). Even though the prevention of pregnancy has always been a part of traditional medical practices in Niger, the idea that contraception is a foreign imposition has emerged forcefully in certain discourses:

> Family planning was imposed on us. Twenty years ago, we didn't know about the pill. Women used products that came from knowledge of our environment. . . . See all the publicity they try to give it; that's proof that it's something they want to integrate into our habits. (MG, 49 years old, traditional healer and provider of contraceptive methods, Lazaret district)

In Niger, where society is characterized by a marked differentiation by sex, the advent of biomedical contraception has given many urban women the opportunity to integrate new models of fertility management into their lives. This is a change, which in one way or another removes the monopoly of social management of reproduction from the family structure, where it was previously embedded. However, this revolution inevitably faces impediments. We are thus going to witness the comingling and confrontation of social and biomedical expectations. Women find themselves at the intersection of multiple social changes and try to navigate through them.

Debates about the positive effects of contraception on the female condition are common, but the fact remains that social constraints considerably slow the spread of biomedical contraception, however irreversible it now appears to be. Angus McLaren observes that "it is easier to understand today that, while it may have a liberating effect on women, a high rate of fertility control does not necessarily mean that women enjoy greater freedom" (1990: 21). Indeed, at this point individual control of fertility is still unimaginable except in a small number of situations that women go to considerable lengths to create. The choices that are thinkable to individuals, according to Mary Douglas, are shaped by the institutions within which they live. Douglas points out that "individuals in crises do not make life-and-death decisions on their own. Who shall be saved and who shall die is settled by institutions" (1986: 4).

Fertility decisions affect not only the life and death of the individual but that of society as a whole. Accordingly, social institutions in Niger privilege a pro-natal impulse. Social norms prohibit contraception and abortion the same way they condemn infertility. Despite extensive campaigns to promote biomedical contraception and despite the resources mobilized by international organizations to this end, the use of contraception is far from being socially acceptable in Niger. More often than not, the use of contraceptive products provokes social, marital, and religious tensions. In a medical setting where contraceptive practice is valued and popularized, the tensions are of a different nature and take the form of confrontation between patients and caregivers.

Religious Debates

Islam is a central point of reference for the average Nigerien. There is a strong anchoring of Muslim practices within the population's habits. While it is important not to obscure the existence of more moderate interpretations of Islam, the religious "fundamentalist" waves that emerged in the early 1990s have expanded across all regions of the country.[1] These Muslim fundamentalists are generally referred to as "Izalists" or "Islamists." The number of Muslim associations has seen exponential growth in recent years. At the beginning of 2006, there were nearly a hundred Muslim associations in the country. Among these, those with Islamist inclinations are the most numerous and vocal (Hassane, Doka, and Makama Bawa 2006).

In some quarters, interpretations of Islam have become extreme, particularly in Maradi, Niger's major economic center bordering Nigeria. In 2005, protests by Islamists temporarily blocked polio vaccinations for children under the pretext that children would be sterilized by the West—the same argument brandished by some to discourage the use of medical contraception. This predisposition to reject Western medicine and practices discourages acceptance of biomedical contraception. Some fundamentalist leaders discourage contraception in any form.

Most politicians feel obligated to cooperate with vocal Islamist groups. Islamists tried to remove the reference to Niger as a secular republic during negotiations on the 1999 Constitution. Important draft laws, such as the

---

1. Editor's note: Salafi influences to return to a "purer" form of Islamic practice were on the rise at the time HM was conducting her study (see Sounaye 2021).

family code, languished on the back burner for years due to an outcry from Islamists. Despite support for the draft family code from many non-sectarian women's groups, Islamist women's groups proclaimed that they were deeply opposed to the code.[2] These associations also adopt a low profile when it comes to discussing the rights of women to access contraception; they have never clearly come out in favor of married women's use of contraceptive methods. In the absence of a family code, a women's association, the Union for the Promotion of Nigerien Women, prepared and submitted to the government a preliminary draft law on marriage and divorce that aimed to be consistent with Islam and favorable to women in 2006. This proposal will not be easily made into law, and even if it is, it will just be another legal text on paper.[3]

In the legislative field, Islamists do not specifically mobilize around the issue of contraception but contest texts deemed to be contrary to Islam, particularly bills relating to the status of women. A bill authorizing the ratification of the African Charter on Human and Peoples' Rights on the Rights of Women, when introduced in the National Assembly during its the final session of 2006, was rejected because of fierce opposition from fundamentalists. This opposition manifested in the form of Islamist associations' organization of marches, rallies, and public protest sermons in Niamey. Inside the assembly room, some parliamentarians openly refused to support it because they deemed it contrary to the principles of Islam.

The 1979 Convention on the Elimination of All Forms of Discrimination Against Women was belatedly ratified by Niger in 1999 during a political transition, a time when contested measures are more easily passed.[4] The ratification, however, was made with many reservations. Shortly after, in June 2000, to address the underrepresentation of women in state structures and, according to some observers, make concrete

---

2. I would argue that reformists created Islamist women's associations (including the Union of Muslim Women in Niger, the Nigerien Association of Muslim Women, and the Jamiyat Nassaratul Dine association, among others) to undermine any proposed emancipation for Nigerien women. As in the Maghreb, patriarchal legal structures depend upon women to uphold patriarchal systems (Lacoste-Dujardin [1985] 1996). Islamists are skilled at creating structures like these that combat women's emancipation by proxy. Editor's note: It is possible that HM was mistaken in including Jamiyat Nassaratul Dine, which to our knowledge did not vocally oppose the draft family code and pursues a different interpretation of Islam than the reformists on this list.

3. Editor's note: HM's prediction that revisions to family law in Niger would be unlikely to succeed proved correct. On the outcome of these struggles, see Kang (2015).

4. Ordinance No. 99-30 of August 13, 1999.

progress toward the emancipation of women, Law No. 2000-008 was signed, establishing a gender quota system. The quota required that a minimum of 25% of appointments to posts in the government and public administration and 10% of candidates on electoral lists go to whichever gender is underrepresented.[5]

Niamey, like Maradi and Zinder, is experiencing a religious "revival." This is reflected by the increased construction of mosques throughout the city, the regular occurrence of public sermons, and the permanent acoustic siege by Muslim preachers on radio and television stations. Veils are more present in everyday life, women (but also men) seek to be more "pious," and aggression (generally verbal) toward those deemed deviant is more common than in the past.

Through conviction or for strategic reasons, many use religious arguments to oppose the use of any contraception for the regulation of fertility. The perception that there is incompatibility between contraception and Islam is so widespread that it dissuades some, including those who would benefit from it, from seeking contraception.

Discussion on the use of coitus interruptus sheds some light on the stance of some Muslim scholars on contraception. In light of this practice (*al asl*) Muslim scholars argue that contraception can be acceptable as long as it does not have harmful effects on the health of the mother or child and as long as it is implemented in a temporary and provisional manner (Djibo et al. 1998). Many religious figures work to prevent public family planning programs from promoting techniques and practices geared toward either the complete cessation of childbearing (such as tubal ligation) or the limitation of the overall number of births, instead encouraging better birth spacing. Such a position acknowledges that sexual activity does not necessarily have to be procreative (Bouhdiba 2001: 118–119; Omran 1992; Nasr 2000).

The most rigid of Niger's Islamist scholars, however, see contraception as contrary to the injunction to increase the number of Muslims. They reiterate the Qur'anic belief that "God feeds every mouth created"; Allah, the provider of sustenance, feeds all. Those Muslims whose reading of contraception is founded on the tradition of *al asl* have begun to push back. The Society of Islamic Associations for Family Planning and Social Development (Groupement des Associations Islamiques en matière de

5. Editor's note: The minimum for electoral lists was raised from 10% to 15% and then 25% in Laws No. 2014-64 and No. 2019-69, respectively. In the 2019 quota reform, the 25% minimum for appointments to government posts was raised to 30%.

Planification Familiale et Développement Sociale [GAIPDS]) was created in 1997 with the financial support of Luxembourg's development cooperation as part of the fight against AIDS and of the United Nations Population Fund (UNFPA) through its Reproductive Health and the Advancement of Women in Islam (Santé de la Reproduction et Promotion de la Femme en Islam) project. The 13 associations that make up this group seek to defend the promotion of family planning in Niger. They introduced a discourse arguing that Islamic values are not fundamentally contrary to the principles of population and reproductive health policy. According to them, it is possible to draw a connection between the Muslim tradition and contemporary public health practices (Moussa Abdallah 2002: 36). As one member of GAIPDS said,

> The use of a given form of contraception, if it does not come from an illicit product or entity, is indeed accepted in Islam. But there are individuals who, for very subjective reasons, disseminate the opposite idea. (Malam AY, Collège Mariama district)

In some neighborhoods in Niamey, such as Boukoki, the hardening of religious practice is visible in the growing practice of confining women to the home.[6] Through this dogmatic interpretation, Islam confers relatively extensive powers on a man in the management of his home, and any movement of a married woman outside the marital home, as well as her economic undertakings, must be subject to the husband's authorization. Islamists and conservative traditionalists argue that, for a married Muslim woman, entry into paradise is conditional upon her strict respect of conjugal rules, a respect that includes providing sexual satisfaction, as well as spiritual and ideological subordination, to her husband. Religion has become a pretext for rejecting contraception for reasons related to finance, jealousy, or authoritarianism. In this framework, a husband's veto is always decisive. A common maxim regularly reminds a woman that her happiness in this world and in the afterlife is to be sought at her husband's feet. The dominance of "religious civil society," combined with present-day social change, reduces both the individual freedoms of women and the state's power to enforce public policies, such as those related to population.

---

6. Editor's note: On seclusion (*kuble or kulle*) and women's agency in accessing space and education in Niger, see Alidou (2005).

Complex Marital and Social "Transactions"

Although having offspring confers a higher status upon both men and women, children in patrilineal societies are generally claimed by men from the husband's lineage, while in matrilineal societies they are claimed by men of the mother's lineage (Andro 2001).

Within a matrimonial home, the husband and wife (or wives) do not always agree on the management of the woman's fertility. Many men want the right to oversee not only their wives' reproductive lives but their health in its entirety:

> Yes, there are men who don't even want their wives to have injections without their permission. But it depends on their individual character. There are even men who prevent access to their homes during mobile vaccination campaigns. You know that in cases like this, a wife can't get to a health center for any reason whatsoever without her husband's blessing. (Madame FM, nurse, integrated health center [*centre de santé intégré* [CSI], Boukoki)

The attitudes and behaviors of men when it comes to contraception are of vital importance, but they have been overlooked in family planning programs (Andro and Hertrich 2001). Such programs neglect the fact that contraception is decided upon and practiced by the couple.

Initially, when the first family planning programs were launched exclusively for married women in the early 1980s, women who came for consultations were required to demonstrate their husband's approval by presenting their husband's ID card. This approach, far from creating the conditions for cooperation between spouses regarding contraception, reinforced notions of men's guardianship over women and often triggered the husband's opposition. Women would then be constrained to "borrow" these precious cards to receive consultations in health centers. Presentations of the proof of identity did not necessarily mean that the husband and wife reached an agreement. Since the formal recognition of a woman's right to contraception in 1988, women have not been required to provide evidence of their husband's approval, facilitating married women's access and opening the way for single women to seek contraception.

Since that time, in both major family planning programs and health centers, reproductive counseling has remained directed solely at women. The provision of medical contraception is almost never a question of counseling the couple. Yet taking pills, inserting an intrauterine device (IUD), and implanting a Norplant are all therapeutic approaches and initiatives that are by no means easy for a woman to undertake whether done in secret or in the most total transparency. This applies to both "individual methods" (pill, IUD, and injections) as well as "cooperative methods" (withdrawal, periodic or prolonged abstinence, and wearing a condom). This one-sided approach to contraception creates a climate of suspicion around married women's movements.

Some men disapprove of all methods of birth control, whether individual or cooperative. The husband generally justifies his refusal to consider contraception by arguing that it is his responsibility as the provider of material and financial means to make such decisions. If men are open to contraception, they are more inclined to use cooperative methods. But still, cooperative methods are little used. Withdrawal and condoms are said to decrease pleasure during sexual intercourse. Abstinence, by reducing sexual activity, undermines the contemporary reading of a Muslim marital couple's sexual duties to one another, according to which regular sexual relations are authorized whenever the husband desires so long as the appropriate conditions of health and religious purity are met.

A woman's use of contraception leads to suspicions of her committing adultery. As I argue throughout this book, because of the strategic importance of reproduction in society, women's sexuality and fertility are subject to strict social surveillance. From the testing of a bride's virginity; throughout pregnancy, childbirth, and breastfeeding; to the weaning of the child, women's private lives are closely monitored. This "voyeurism" on the part of the extended family responds to the concern over the perpetuation of the group in accordance with its rules. When a woman uses contraceptives despite strong opposition from her husband, she is sometimes accused of having adulterous relationships by her husband or by her in-laws. This generates problems of trust within the matrimonial home.

Medical contraception is perceived very negatively. Rightly or wrongly, it is thought that a woman who uses it without her husband's knowledge or against his will might have a penchant for sexual profligacy. I had three closely spaced pregnancies that were very difficult. I suggested contraception to my husband. He replied that he didn't want to use any medical contraceptives but that we could practice abstinence while I was ovulating. We tried to do that for four months. In the end, my husband didn't keep his promise, and I reminded him about it. He simply told me that it didn't matter because the children who would be born would be under his care and he can afford it. But me, I didn't agree. That's when I started secretly going to a PMI [maternal and infant health services clinic (*protection maternelle et infantile*)] where a midwife friend works. Unfortunately, someone told my husband about my trips to the medical center. I'm sure it was one of his sisters. I ran into a friend of hers at the PMI. As a result, he found contraceptives in the drawers of the bed that I had forgotten to hide. . . . It went very badly, because my husband decided that if I took this medication despite his opposition, it must be because I was hiding something from him. You see, he thought this something was a lover. It was so humiliating for me. What's more, his family supported him. We got into such a fight that I had to go to my parents. I stayed at their house for 82 days. We really almost divorced. We are barely reconciled. I got pregnant soon after going back. And since I just can't take any more of these repeated deliveries. . . . Can you imagine? Four kids in less than eight years of marriage. I just can't take it anymore and I know this problem will come up again. I need contraception, but my husband still doesn't want to hear anything about it. The most important thing in a couple is trust, but that's gone between us. (Madame H née NH, 30 years old, four children, ministry official, Boukoki district)

Crises of confidence surrounding contraceptive use are not specific to Niger and are found elsewhere in Africa. In Senegal, for example, men equate contraception to women's sexual liberation, even refusing to allow their wives to use contraception for the spacing of births (Wade 2001: 269). Similarly, among the Yoruba of Nigeria, Koster writes, "the distrust of his wife's fidelity (sound or not) may cause a husband to forbid her to use modern contraceptives" (2003: 305). Some women believe men raise the specter of infidelity as a pretext for them to argue against biomedical contraception. So long as conditions for marital dialog are missing, there can be no real negotiation around sexual and reproductive health. Yet in many African couples, open discussion of such questions is taboo (Omondi-Odhiambo 1997; Sala-Diakanda and Kassegne 2001). Even among educated couples, these issues are barely discussed (Lutz-Fuchs 1994). To improve the legitimacy of a contraceptive technique, the relational dimension of fertility management must not be neglected (Andro 2001; Andro and Hertrich 2001; Moussa Abdallah 2002).[7]

Most questions related to the marital couple (sexuality, birth control, and male–female relationships) are socially managed by the man's and the woman's respective family groups. The influence of the husband's group is stronger, if not exclusive, since the wife's subordination in marriage places her in a secondary role relative to her in-laws.

7. Editor's note: Since 2008 the UNFPA and the Nigerien Ministry of Public Health have worked together to promote a program to educate married men in groups known as École des Maris or "Husbands' school" on family planning methods and the advantages of birth spacing—this initiative has been remarkably popular. HM had a role in bringing this program into being. It nevertheless struggles without sufficient funding.

As soon as you get married, your in-laws are immediately concerned about the children you're going to have. They're much more interested in that than anything else. You've barely given birth, and they start asking about more. When you want to do family planning, even with your husband's agreement, they can veto it. The husband's parents consider your children as property that belongs to them that they can remove from your guardianship at any time and at their discretion. As a result, a widow faces many problems determining her children's education or future, simply because the brother, uncle, or mother of her late husband has already claimed all rights in the matter. (Madame FK, 31 years old, woman giving birth, PMI Gaweye)

As one interviewee underscores, family pressure can be exerted on both women and men. There are couples, certainly few in number, who collaborate to determine their fertility and family life but who find themselves confronted by their extended families and their respective parents. Couples experience this control especially acutely if they live in the "big house" of an extended family.

Women are closely monitored in the concessions where several households live. Even when your brother visits, all it takes is for one or two people not to recognize him for suspicions to spread. When you leave the house your husband's brothers, sisters, or cousins always arrange to accompany you, because you're not always trusted. In the street, even when you're alone, you have to know who to talk to. Otherwise, from simple misunderstandings, people can cause serious problems in your home life. (Madame OH, 34 years old, six children, housewife, Gaweye district)

Nevertheless, Armelle Andro goes too far when she generalizes that in West Africa "relationships between married men and women take place, in a way, outside of the couple." Andro states that, "[t]he very notion of a conjugal unit really has, at least for the great majority of the population, neither a sociological reality nor a psychological reality" (2001: 76). While it is true that the couple faces pressure from relatives, this conclusion has an ethnocentric bias, common among researchers who examine other societies through the lens of their own. The relational and affective aspects of a couple's life are matters of individual experience and luck.

The housewife, in addition to her economic dependence upon others, is socially assigned the role of child bearer. Moreover, the high priority that women themselves give to motherhood in their personal and familial trajectories can overshadow the interventions of outsiders and husbands. Because it is unlikely that a woman will be able to negotiate her reproductive destiny, women themselves internalize these same constraints. The rhythms of reproduction are then experienced by women as a form of self-constraint. The difficulty in establishing the line between an external imposition and willing compliance is also due to the fact that women sometimes inflict upon themselves constraints beyond those imposed externally. In some cases, they require more of themselves than any outside force. As Bozon writes, "the symbolic violence of a woman's duty to reproduce in very fertile societies comes from the fact that they can't not desire many children" (2001: 176). Unlike "emancipated" Western women, these women do not develop a "plan" to have children but rather accept motherhood as their destiny, one they also know is rarely negotiable. Even though some women seek to space their births, few are likely to specify how many children they will have. When asked in interviews, people almost always leave the ceiling undefined:

> We happily accept the number of children God wants to give. (HD, 26 years old, father of one child, launderer, Boukoki district)

In general, women ask for the maximum possible, showing that they are perfectly in line with society's voracious demands. Besides, for many people, daring to project into the future in such a calculated way amounts to succumbing to "the White mentality of wanting to control everything."

> We can't say in advance how many children we want. You don't even know what your life will be like tomorrow. It's God who decides these things. (HD, 26 years old, father of one child, launderer, Boukoki district)

Notwithstanding this omnipresent authority held by the husband in addition to the interference of familial networks in the regulation of procreation, women do deploy microstrategies of evasion and circumvention that enable them to conceal their actions. I turn to these next.

MANIPULATING SOCIAL RULES: EVIDENCE OF WOMEN'S COUNTERVAILING AGENCY

Social rules, however severe, are not inviolable. Individuals, either alone or in association with others, have always developed strategies enabling them to evade social control. This is particularly true of those whose power has little recognition in the public social space. In this section, I will identify some of the maneuvers women described in interviews to thwart the social rules imposed by men, society, and kinship groups. In local phraseology, such microstrategies are referred to as *woyboro dabari* (Z) or *dubaarun maata* (H) (women's clever tricks, women's arts, feminine shrewdness). Like Sylvie Fainzang (1991: 104), I have identified in my own research a variety of schemes used by women to circumvent the conjugal debt of reproductive sexuality in exchange for upkeep: illness, fake menstruation, fatigue, and, more unusually, sex strikes or sexual blackmail.

When women feign illness, they may invoke either emotional or physical pain. They therefore place their husbands in the position of making the decision to abstain from sex. As Madame RA (25 years old, one child, education volunteer, Say Department) said to me,

> Of course, it's a grave sin for a woman to refuse to her husband, but one can always feign illness so as not to commit *sunna*.

A woman may initially invoke sadness (*bini hasarow* [Z]) to explain her inability to pay the conjugal debt that she sometimes finds unwelcome. Nevertheless, some respondents say this trick is less successful than conjuring up an imaginary physical illness because some men distinguish between mental and physical indisposition. For them, sadness or melancholy has no bearing on the obligations of the marital sexual relationship. In line with this idea, Madame ZM said that,

> Sometimes when you tell your husband you have *bini hasarow*, he might tell you that has nothing to do with what he's asking you to do. (29 years old, four children, housewife, Collège Mariama district)

However, sexual invitations are rarely made in cases where this sadness is related to bereavement or another unfortunate event that has occurred within one's entourage or that of the spouse.

As for faking physical illness, this might range from headaches (*bon doori* [Z]) to stomachaches (*gunde doori*), including lower back pain (*banda doori*), dizziness (*mo binni*), and palpitations (*bini doori*). Whatever the false symptom, it serves to forestall repaying the conjugal debt while avoiding a direct confrontation (Shorter 1984, referenced in Fainzang 1991).

Claiming to be menstruating is the most common trick women use to evade their sexual duty. Madame RA also said to me,

> I especially do it while I'm ovulating. If I don't, I risk getting pregnant. I gave birth just last year. It's all I can do since I can't practice contraception the way I want.

Men often have little understanding of their wives' menstrual cycles, which women can manipulate as they please. Muslim women must not say their prayers during menstruation. The observation of women's ablutions and prayers is generally the only indication that men have of ensuring their "sexual availability."

> For almost all women, menstruation is our little trick. Even if a man is poorly educated, he wouldn't dare check that there's blood flowing from you. The only means they have to verify our cycle is our prayer times, and nothing more. Many men don't know how to calculate the rest. (Madame SI, 35 years old, five children, sanitation worker, Niamey Municipality V)

The ruse therefore consists of saying prayers out of the husband's sight and improvising frequent washing of underwear.

The pretext of fatigue functions in the same way as that of illness. A wife counters her husband's wishes with her physical inability to perform the sexual act.

> You can pretend to be very tired. You show your husband that you're not "*opérationnel.*" It annoys some men when their wives aren't dynamic during sex. (Madame HB3, 26 years old, two children, housewife, Niamey)

Nevertheless, feigning fatigue does not always achieve the expected objectives. Some men continue to seek their satisfaction, ignoring this limitation. As one woman remarked,

> For some men, the essential is that they ejaculate, and they often don't care what the context is. (Madame BH, 33 years old, five children, grocer, Lamordé district)

In the context of polygamy, sexual activity can amount to open warfare (Fainzang and Journet 2002). Togolese novelist and essayist Sami Tchak observes that both women and men engage in sexual blackmail.

> Sex is indeed a weapon within couples, a weapon that husbands and wives employ along with all manner of trickery: to wean a wife from her sexual rations to punish her for a disobedience, to subordinate her, to obtain from her what she would not have agreed upon otherwise; to deny a husband the secret passageways of the body to get something from him, etc. (1999: 41)

Indeed, among all the forms of resistance shown by women, this form of protest is the most successful in the sense that the insubordination is in no way concealed or feigned. In these cases, women, without supplying reasons such as illness, menstruation, or sadness, simply refuse to submit to their conjugal duty. My research suggests, however, that the use of blackmail is not widespread. A Muslim woman who commits sexual blackmail puts herself in a position of sinning twice over: by refusing the sexual act and by disobeying her husband.

CONTRACEPTIVE SUBVERSION

For some respondents, a woman's mastery of contraception can subvert men's power over the management of fertility. Women may act alone or with the support of accomplices who are family relations or who live nearby. First, women have devised tricks to escape the surveillance of their husbands and the husbands' families to go to healthcare facilities for reproductive and contraceptive consultations. This is easier for women whose husbands spend a lot of time outside the home.

> Personally, I've been taking pills secretly for four years. My husband is surprised we haven't had a new baby for three years. I told him it's related to his travels; that I'm always ovulating while he's away. It's not very convincing, is it? He suspects something but can't prove anything. (Madame BO, 33 years old, four children, housewife, Goudel district)

A woman's medical file, which she must bring with her when she goes to the clinic, bears the evidence of the use of medical contraception. For women whose husbands are both literate and opposed to contraceptive practice, the trick is to entrust the consultation book to a relative, friend, or neighbor in solidarity with the cause. The file is a piece of evidence that women are careful not to leave lying around because its discovery can result in marital tensions.

> I've been using family planning for almost two and a half years, but my husband doesn't know. After the birth of my third child, and before he became an Izalist, we had talked about the possibility of using the pill to space my pregnancies. But now he doesn't want to hear any of it because he thinks it's going against God's will. So I take advantage of his absences to go to the clinic. The midwife always gives me a three-month supply of pills so I don't have to go every month

and arouse my husband's suspicion. After I go to the center, I leave my file with my cousin. To keep him from suspecting anything, I recently faked a miscarriage and he believed it. (Madame HB4, 28 years old, telephone card seller, Boukoki district)

Women often arrange to carry out family planning consultations and obtain contraception under the pretext of seeking other medical services. Some women confided that they took the opportunity to kill two birds with one stone whenever they sought out curative consultations for adult ailments (malaria, migraines, colic, or colds, to name a few) or for consultations for their children. To attend a family planning appointment, a woman might invent a discomfort or illness for her child, who she must take to the CSI. In other cases, some women also invent the illness of a loved one (parents, friends, or colleagues) to go to the maternity ward or PMI center.

All means are used to deceive husbands. All women have a whole range of *dubaarun maata* ("women's clever tricks" [H]). There are a lot of things you can invent to slip away from your husband's surveillance. Most often, I invent friends who are giving birth or who are sick, in addition to making up fake appointments. (Madame SK, 32 years old, one child, housewife, Kirkissoye district)

Women who use the pill may engage in "consultation by proxy." Some midwives and attendants are also involved in this game of proxy consultation. They often take on the role of intermediary between the health structures that employ them and the friends, relatives, or neighbors who need their services. Here, a woman sends people from her entourage to go to an appointment in her place:

I go to the center when I can manage to escape the surveillance of my in-laws. When that's not possible, my neighbor who's a room attendant gets the medicine for me. (Madame BO, 33 years old, housewife, Goudel district)

Ideally, a woman takes care to provide her stand-in the date of her last period and her obstetric history. If she fails to do so, she may receive contraceptives that do not match her gynecological profile or menstrual cycle.

For women across the socioeconomic spectrum, the itinerant sale of pharmaceutical products can be invaluable. Because the vendors come directly to the home and carry products for a host of ailments, they ensure a level of discretion that is difficult to find in health centers or in formal pharmacies. Approached for countless ailments, itinerant pharmacists are often part of the network of "accomplices" of women taking contraception.

> Before, I used to fake headaches, stomachaches, or anything to see the "pill seller" (*kini koyo* [Z]). Now that we've known each other for a long time—a year and a half—I've reached an agreement with one so he brings me pills at the end of each month. He comes when my husband goes to the market for his daily activities. Often, he watches for him to leave. He even brings pills for friends of mine who fear being discovered by their husbands or in-laws. (Madame HB5, 29 years old, four children, knitter, Gaweye district)

The use of street pharmacies, like consultation by proxy, only concerns oral contraception. With modest means, a woman can implement a contraceptive practice in her married life despite opposition from her husband. These choices reduce the risk of tension and interference from the rest of the extended family.

Generally, women who can manage to do so prefer injectable contraception because of the relatively limited constraints associated with their use.

> I took the pill for five months, but at what cost! I changed their hiding place every day until the day my husband finally saw them. I had to lie to him, telling him it was for my sister, and that she was coming to get them. It worked because it was a new pack I hadn't started yet. . . . After that day, I decided to change my method according to advice from the same sister. Now they give me the injection and I don't really have any issues. Arranging to go to the PMI once every three months is very easy. (Madame SK, 32 years old, one child, housewife, Kirkissoye district)

While pill packs and the accompanying documentation must be brought into the home and hidden, this is not the case with injections. All the secrecy of contraceptive practice remains between the walls of the PMI or the maternity center (if, of course, the personnel remain discreet).

Thus, women's microstrategies are deployed to introduce contraception into a couple's sexual life against the wishes of the husband or in-laws. There are also situations where men are worried about their excess fertility and impose contraception on their wives. This is particularly the case in polygamous environments where the complex power relationships between co-wives are closely managed. In these instances, women may attempt to improve their chances of becoming pregnant and avoid the contraceptive practices endorsed by their husbands.

MATRIMONIAL STRATEGIES AND CONTRACEPTIVE PRACTICE

Not all women seek to space their births. In some monogamous households, women seek closely spaced births to attain a strategic position within the conjugal space. A woman who hopes to discourage her partner from taking another wife may scheme to become pregnant. The presence in the household of numerous offspring offers a safeguard of the interests of the wife and her children. We thus find women who stay in the matrimonial home only because of their numerous offspring, the love between them and their husbands having been gone for a very long time:

> My older sister and her husband haven't been on good terms for a long time now. But what do you expect—with seven children on her arms, where can she go, and besides, who would want her? She continues to live under the marital roof because of her children. When her fourth child was born, her husband wanted her to start contraception, but she refused and continued to give birth at very close intervals. She doesn't dare leave. Nor does her husband have the courage to chase her away. But he's already taken a new wife. She's young and he only cares for her. He does provide food and often clothing for my sister. (Madame BH, 28 years old, teacher, Yantala district)

The "child pretext" therefore can prevent the marital tie from breaking definitively and may ensure that a languishing marriage survives for better or worse.

Inside polygamous homes, rivalry between co-wives is often expressed through childbearing. Fertility, or at least superior childbearing, is a strategy developed by each of the co-wives to attain the "preferred" status with their spouse. According to Fainzang and Journet, "the dominant idea is that it is through giving children that a wife preserves the affection and favors of her husband" (2002: 221). The competitive ideology of motherhood in society in general, but more particularly in polygamous spaces, constitutes a major obstacle to contraceptive practice in all its forms. Thus, "the rivalry between co-wives makes the intrusion of contraception more problematic in polygamous environments than in monogamous environments" (2002: 223).

In this constant race for motherhood, there is little likelihood that contraception will be used, even when the husband is favorable to it. In a society where the majority of men are opposed to the use of contraceptive products, occasionally it is the husband who wants to limit births. It is easier for a woman who wants to use contraception without her husband's consent to accomplish her aim to avoid pregnancy than it is for a man to impose contraception upon his wife against her will. One woman who has strategically stopped using the pill (which she had taken previously with her husband's consent) upon the arrival of a second wife into her home, said,

> In five years of marriage, I found myself with two children on my arms and a pregnancy to manage. I wanted to stop this disaster (*hasaraw* [Z]), but I also feared my husband's reaction. I never would have guessed that he would be the one to ask me, as my delivery approached, to opt to start contraception immediately after the birth of our child. . . . So I used contraception for 32 months before contracting my fourth pregnancy. After that one was born, I continued using it. . . . But in the meantime, he's married again and his new wife doesn't use contraception. She's made it clear to those close to her that she never will. You see? She wants to catch up with the number of children I have. So what do you think I'm going to do? I've stopped using contraception. Now our sisters-in-law often make jokes to our husband that "there's a baptism at our house every year." In 12 years of marriage, I had five children, while in six years, she's already had three. You must understand that I can't put myself in a bad position. Our husband has mentioned this to us on several occasions. For now, he leaves us alone, but I know he's just putting up with it. Maybe he'll take action in due course. (Madame ZK, 31 years old, five children, ministry official, Zabarkan district)

Contrary to the assumption in much of the literature that a woman in a monogamous household is likely to have more children than a woman in a polygamous household, my research suggests a more complicated picture. In my interviews, women in monogamous households generally did observe postpartum sexual abstinence during the 40 days after birth and often during breastfeeding. Even if these prescriptions are less rigorously respected than in the past, the fact remains that they generally favor a "natural" spacing of births, which can also be deliberately reinforced by employing contraception. Indeed, it is more likely that women in monogamous households will consider adopting a given contraceptive method. By contrast, the competitive environment between co-wives produces attitudes unfavorable to any form of contraceptive practice, including postpartum abstinence. Prohibitions are not respected because each wife wants to get pregnant again quickly. For each of them, it is a question of minimizing their risk of divorce by developing ways to perpetuate their presence in the matrimonial home. A mother is thereby able to increase the share of inheritance that goes to her own children rather than to her co-wife's.

The "sexual and reproductive rivalries" highlighted by Fainzang (1991: 100) undermine contraception in a polygamous environment. The system of "turns" through which a husband must share the bed of each of his wives equally in rotation has no significant contraceptive effect on an individual woman's fertility. However, if he cheats by going to both wives on the same day, he violates the sacred contractual balance of polygamy in Islam:

> Not all men fear God. Many don't hesitate to bring debauchery into their own homes. God said to divide the number of days spent with each wife evenly and fairly. Instead, many steal (*i ga zay no* [Z]). It's the equivalent of adultery. (Madame HB5, 29 years old, four children, knitter, Gaweye district)

Polygamous men whose children are baptized only a few days apart are sometimes suspected of having cheated. It is acknowledged, however, that two wives whose ovulatory cycles are one to three days apart can become pregnant at almost the same time without their husband needing to "cheat"; each wife has her turn every 48 hours and, in some cases, every 24 hours. The height of these rumors is reached when, in extremely rare cases, two co-wives give birth on the same day. This logically implies the simultaneous organization of two baptisms for the husband, who is at this time subject to much criticism and feelings of great embarrassment (Fainzang 1991: 95; Fainzang and Journet 1989, 2002).

> If a woman gets pregnant on a day that's not her turn, the unborn child is considered a *zinaizé* (Z)—the equivalent of a bastard. Her child is illegitimate. (Madame HB5, 29 years old, four children, knitter, Gaweye district)

Fainzang sums up this dynamic: "the wives of polygamists are thus the perpetuators of the system that has assigned them to reproduction. Although the foundations of natalist ideology tend to have less of a stronghold in urban areas, the maximization of procreation remains the goal of women in polygamous homes" (1991: 100).

CONCLUSION

Fatima Mernissi refers to the artifices that women use to subvert the social order as *kayd* (Arabic), "the power to deceive and defeat men through cunning and intrigue" (quoted by Lacoste-Dujardin [1985] 1996: 95). How should we characterize the microstrategies women use to temporarily evade engaging in sex or to use biomedical contraception on the sly? I agree with Fainzang and Journet, who conclude, "while claiming illness permits a woman to escape, at least temporarily, sexual obligations in marriage, such pretexts don't amount to real resistance because they don't challenge the injunction to obey her husband and they contribute to the reproduction of unequal sexual relations" (2002: 223).

The diversity of contraceptive methods explored in the preceding chapter reveals that a woman's desire to have a child does not preclude a desire to regulate her pregnancies. Furthermore, the expectation to reproduce exists alongside the stigmatization of closely grouped births. Medical contraceptive use might be higher if women felt more comfortable or in control (Jaffré 1999). Whether a woman puts herself on contraception without her husband's knowledge or, as I shall discuss in the following chapter, she seeks out an abortion, these are signs of a counter-hegemonic impulse that is not visible in the public sphere. They occupy the limited space women have to negotiate freedom in the face of a dominating force they cannot openly confront.

By succeeding in dodging what Bouhdiba (2001) calls the "pious obligation," the conjugal debt, a woman gains, if only temporarily, some modest ground in the marital contest. Yet, aside from sexual blackmail, which is the most daring form of protest, women usually employ subtle ruses to evade the grip of men and social or religious rules. The most commonly employed tactics to circumvent and combat the power and domination of men, however, often contribute to the reinforcement of women's dependency.

CHAPTER 8

The Realities of Abortion

In the city of Niamey, the use of abortion as a method of contraception was reported by many respondents. It is generally thought that this practice only concerns unmarried women: young girls, widows, and divorced women. However, studies show that married women should not be left out of the discussion (Moumouni 2000: 107). Whether inside or outside marriage there are affective, marital, social, economic, and medical considerations that push women to have an abortion (Moussa Abdallah 2002). Abortion constitutes a form of what I refer to as "infertile sexuality" because a potential birth is "prohibited" (Bologne 1988). While recourse to abortion is a fairly widespread phenomenon in Niamey and concerns women from all walks of life, its scope is difficult to measure. Its importance surely varies from one social group to another. For married women, the group that I am particularly interested in, it is relatively easy to pass an abortion off as a miscarriage.

A methodological remark should be made here. The wide range of abortive methods and products in evidence in my field research proves that abortions are common but are largely invisible in the surrounding environment for reasons of secrecy. Indeed, despite the numerous forms of specialized knowledge and customs in evidence, it was impossible for me to obtain certain details on the practices used in inducing abortions. While interviews provide some insights, ideally, we would seek out first-hand witnesses, persuade a medical practitioner or therapeutic specialist to speak up, or somehow otherwise pierce the secrecy surrounding abortive procedures. Like the act of adultery, which also remains obstinately

Yearning and Refusal. Hadiza Moussa, Edited by Alice J. Kang and Barbara M. Cooper, Oxford University Press.
© Oxford University Press 2023. DOI: 10.1093/oso/9780197662113.003.0009

hidden, abortion is kept secret by those who have them and by their accomplices.[1]

First, I address the connections that might exist between the use of contraception and the use of abortion. Then, I explore some of the circumstances in which unmarried and married women might seek abortion and discuss whether abortion is a way of contesting the social order. I then outline the legal barriers, the social and religious criticism of abortion, and popular Zarma and Hausa phraseology surrounding abortion in the Nigerien environment. Without claiming to be exhaustive, I describe known abortive practices in Niamey and finally conclude by connecting the realities of abortion to the concept of infertile sexuality.

CONTRACEPTION AND ABORTION: A CONTINUUM?

Despite the tendency to dissociate contraception and abortion, the two practices generally go hand in hand. In many cases, these processes are inextricably linked as both are intended to promote the return of menstruation, and sometimes one might be used as a substitute for the other.[2] In his history of contraception in Europe, Angus McLaren observes, "Early twentieth-century birth controllers, partly for tactical purposes, attempted to draw a clear line between contraception and abortion. But much of the evidence suggests that women traditionally viewed both as located on a continuum of fertility-regulating strategies" (1990: 8). In Niamey, abortion is most often an enterprise undertaken by women alone, particularly if they are married. In general, married women rarely seek accomplices to direct them toward the "closed circuit" of the termination of pregnancy or to provide them directly with abortive products.

Often, women (married or not) seek an abortion without ever having used biomedical contraception because it is so hard to obtain. Abortion is

---

1. Editor's note: Sounaye, Diarra, and Younoussi (2017) subsequently synthesized the work on abortion done by LASDEL researchers, offering a nuanced picture of abortion as sometimes emerging out of the social negotiation prompted by an unexpected pregnancy. Particularly for single women, an abortion may result from the vision of the future that emerges in light of those negotiations.

2. Editor's note: While it is true that emmenagogues and abortifacients can have the same effect—they can produce the resumption of menstruation—it is not quite accurate to say that contraception in general produces the "return" of menstruation. It is possible to take the pill to avoid menstruation altogether—this is particularly true for athletes and women who have painful periods. Some Muslim women use the pill to prevent menstruation during the hajj.

their contraception. The aim is to refuse to give birth (or at least to postpone it).

> Many young girls and women don't bother coming to health centers or even pharmacies to purchase contraceptives. They simply wait until they get pregnant, then they take action to suppress it. To put it bluntly, they prefer the "curative" properties of abortion over the preventive properties of contraception. For these women, aborting is synonymous with spacing out their births. . . . Some women fail in their attempts at abortion, and they can often be tragic experiences. With contraception, they wouldn't have gone through so much and they wouldn't have taken unnecessary risks. (Midwife, Central Maternity Ward)

Rather than seeing contraception and abortion on a continuum of reproductive control, women in some cases see them as having the same practical value and meaning: abortion is equivalent to contraception. One can thus resort to abortion or contraception interchangeably to regulate one's fertility. One woman who swears she has never attempted an abortion told me this:

> When you have the opportunity to take contraceptives, you do. Otherwise you can have an abortion in the first weeks of pregnancy. It all comes down to the same thing. The main thing is to not carry an unwanted pregnancy. (Madame KM, 34 years old, five children, city official, Niamey)

Similarly, Mariatou Koné reports that in Yopougon and Koumassi (Côte d'Ivoire), "abortion is considered as a contraceptive practice by the female population (and even some men)" (2000: 104). The questions of contraception and of abortion are closely intertwined. Nevertheless, as we will see later in this chapter, the choice to pursue abortion instead of preventive contraceptive methods can also be related to women's difficulty in negotiating with their sexual partners (Guillaume 2009).

ABORTION IN AND OUTSIDE OF MARRIAGE

Because abortion is illegal in Niger, there are no reliable medical statistics on its prevalence, although according to one nurse I spoke to abortion is widespread in Niamey. Officially, medical personnel are only engaged with managing the side effects of an abortion. Even where abortion is legal, it can be difficult to study because it is secretive. Writing about the case of France, sociologist Luc Boltanski explains, "This discretion is precisely what makes abortion difficult to study, not only because anthropological and historical works focused on it are sparse and laconic, but also because, in contemporary societies where abortion is legal, those who have experienced it often prove reluctant to speak about it, even to a 'sociologist' who promises them anonymity" ([2004] 2013: 21). Even in a conjugal context, where one could assume that the failure of a pregnancy was a miscarriage, the researcher can be confronted with almost total silence on the subject. If at first glance both "abortion" and "miscarriage" are interrupted pregnancies, the first results from a deliberate act, while the second occurs spontaneously (Houel and Lhomond 1982).[3] The local lexicon carves out a way to distinguish between different kinds of abortions. In Niger, judgments about an abortion, while generally negative, vary according to the marital status of the individual who has one.

Abortion in a Pre- and Extra-marital Context

Abortions outside of marriage concern secondary school students (middle and high school), young women in higher education, and other single women:

> We often receive cases due to complications of abortions. These are young girls who tried to get rid of an unwanted pregnancy in secret, but who put their lives at risk. They are brought to us here in bad shape and we are required to refer them [to the Central Hospital]. (Midwife, Boukoki Maternity Ward)

The association of abortion with schoolgirls does not mean that other women are exempt from having one. The stakes of pregnancy, however, are particularly high for schoolgirls. In addition to facing social stigma, the difficulty of pursuing both a "maternal career" and a course of study prompts those in school to resort to abortion. Under President Seyni Kountché (1974–1987), any girl in primary or secondary school who became pregnant was expelled, while the person who had impregnated her was brought before the courts. Nowadays, anecdotes about female students who have attempted to or succeeded in disposing an embryo or fetus in campus

---

3. Editor's note: In French the "interruption" of a pregnancy (*avortement*) can be either spontaneous or provoked. In English we would refer to a "spontaneous abortion" as a miscarriage and a "provoked abortion" as an abortion. The close kinship between miscarriage and abortion is preserved in French, as well as the potential ambiguity over the cause of the loss of a pregnancy.

toilets often make news at their schools. Many unmarried girls in this situation want to shelter themselves as much as possible from the social stigma against pregnancy outside marriage. For them the end justifies the means; they go to great lengths to ward off the risks and the social and psychological costs of a pregnancy. Their male partners sometimes cover the cost of the abortion.

Unlike married women who generally receive support from at least part of society (legislation, the medical community, all or part of their entourage), young women are unofficially excluded from accessing contraceptives, both traditional and medical. Many healthcare personnel, reflecting the moral environment surrounding them in Niger, oppose either openly or in private the use of contraception by unmarried women. To avoid providing young women with contraception, medical professionals deploy various dissuasive maneuvers (see Moussa Abdallah 2002; Moussa 2003). Young girls requesting contraception in maternal health centers are often insulted or even reported to their parents by nurses. The expectation elsewhere in the world that single women who are or hope to become professionals will use contraception (Bajos and Ferrand 2004) is subverted by social norms in Niger. In local thinking, contraceptive use is not justified in their case because they are not recognized as having the right to engage in sexual activity.

Under the circumstances, sociologist of religion François-André Isambert explains, "the condemnation of abortion is not solely due to its destructive character, but also because it belongs to the domain of sexuality. Murder [is] bad, but abortion is a source of shame. Its most frequent manifestation ascribes it to a chain of underground sexuality, ranging from illegitimate relationships to single motherhood, from which one seeks to escape" (1982: 367). Agnès Guillaume points out that abortion is not just a family planning issue; it is part of a broader set of concerns that affect the future professional and marital trajectories of single people. Abortion "raises the question of recognizing young women's sexuality. Births outside marriage are often socially condemned, and because access to prevention is difficult or impossible, abortion is sometimes the only possibility for an unmarried woman to avoid a pregnancy that could compromise her future" (2009: 3).

Abortion in a Conjugal Context

Single women are not the only ones who seek abortion; married women also have them. I was able to gain the confidence of some married women who have had an abortion. I will analyze the reasons presented by married women for having an abortion and the logic behind their actions.

The first reflex of women who are married and have an abortion is to call it a miscarriage. In such cases, some married women insist that their pregnancy terminated spontaneously. But among intimates they offer the real reasons for the "miscarriage." Sometimes, in the context of a confidential medical consultation, women explain an abortion as the solution to the failure of or rejection of contraception.

In Niamey, respondents offered a variety of reasons for abortions among married women, some more convincing than others. They might say it was the result of the failure of contraception or that they could not afford or access biomedical contraception. In addition to these reasons, married woman might resort to abortion, as Annik Houel and Brigitte Lhomond put it, "to safeguard an existing or future family happiness" (1982: 498). For a woman who has already given proof of her fertility through the birth of one or more children, abortion offers a means of controlling her fertility following the failure of contraception:

> I was taking the pill, but I sometimes forgot to take it. Even though I usually made up for it by taking the number of missed tablets, apparently this didn't solve the problem because I became pregnant. At first, I thought it was just a late period. I figured it out after two months because I was starting to have dizzy spells and vomiting. That was when I made the decision to abort. My child is only eight months old. It's too early to have another one. (Madame FM, 33 years old, five children, beignet seller, Poudrière district)

Some women mention financial difficulties to explain their non-use of a contraceptive method. The cost of an abortion or to purchase abortive substances, however, is significantly higher than the cost of contraceptives. While a pack of pills costs between 300 and 1,000 CFA francs, an abortion performed by an outside party (a popular specialist or a health professional) can range from 10,000 to 40,000 CFA francs.[4] The financial obstacle to obtaining medical contraception as an account of why a woman has an abortion is not altogether compelling.

A more compelling impediment to regular contraceptive use, perhaps, is the distance of health centers from some women's homes. Women who invoke distance are not all faced with real problems of accessibility, but

4. Editor's note: In 2005, when HM was doing fieldwork for this project, 10,000 CFA francs was roughly $20, and 40,000 CFA francs was close to $80, a major expense when the GDP per capita was $770.

this explanation draws attention to the reality of women's limited access to medical contraception. Close proximity to health centers makes it easier for women to hide contraceptive use from husbands who are opposed to it. Distance from a clinic entails finding the cost of transportation and accounting for prolonged absence from the marital home, which can arouse a husband's suspicions. I have noticed that women who live far from health centers rarely venture to them when they do not have their husband's approval. In short, the closer a woman is to a facility, the easier it is to go there with or without her husband's permission.

> When the health center is near your home, it's easier to go for your consultations. Generally, when it's just renewing a prescription, it doesn't take long at all. Some staff members will serve you right away. Before, I lived far from the women's health clinic and had a lot of trouble getting to my appointments. (Madame FM, 33 years old, five children, beignet seller, Poudrière district)

Another, more social, argument was also brought up by married women. They invoked structural reasons for finding contraceptive access difficult. These related to the operation of health centers, commonly including unpleasant interactions with nursing staff .

Nevertheless, in my own research, I have found that abortion is increasingly used as a contraceptive (Moussa Abdallah 2002: 108). Abortion is a solution to an unplanned or unwanted pregnancy and therefore constitutes "emergency contraception" (Guillaume 2009: 16).

ABORTION: A SIGN OF RESISTANCE TO THE SOCIAL ORDER?

Apart from abortions following a contraceptive practice that has failed, some women have an abortion to show their own kind of resistance to certain social orders: forced marriage, the expectation of producing children, the husband's authority, or the coming of a new co-wife. Women who have not been able to escape forced marriage engage in various forms of resistance, including refusing to give validation to an unwanted union by providing descendants; in other words, they may feign sterility. By way of successive abortions (clandestine, of course), these women manufacture evidence of infertility. By doing so, some of them end up breaking the bonds of their marriage, and then they reconnect with freely chosen partners. Motherhood is thus postponed while they seek out the conjugal relationships that they dreamed of for themselves. Sometimes, women in these circumstances seek abortions after contraceptive failure.

For example, Madame FSH, an unemployed woman of modest elementary schooling, was forced to marry one of her cousins, whom she says she hates (*a ga ay dukurandi no* [Z]). When her longtime boyfriend came forward to make a proposal of marriage he was turned away by the family. Madame FSH married another man but remained in contact with her boyfriend. Having always hoped to marry him, she secretly started taking contraceptives. However, she found it very difficult to take pills regularly. After five months of marriage, she became pregnant. She terminated the pregnancy two months later using noxious products. I met her at the health center following complications resulting from a second abortion. She had been three and a half months along when she took a decoction that one of her friends had procured for her.

Women who simply seek to control their fertility, not escape a marriage, are not quite in the same situation. They are already mothers of several children, and they most often want to space or limit their births. They use abortion as a contraceptive technique for birth spacing or cessation.

> I'm 39 years old and the mother of six children. I would love to take contraception, but my husband is still opposed. Even in my family, no one really supports me aside from one of my aunts. So, I decided to abort. In fact, this is my second abortion. Since my fourth delivery, I've endured enormous pain. I discussed this problem with my husband, but he simply replied: "God is great." I know God is great, but my suffering has not gone away. I don't want to have any more children. I believe I'm sufficiently fulfilled in that regard. But my husband suspects that I don't want to be pregnant anymore because he once told me that he'd bring in another woman who would give him children without resistance. This blackmail means nothing to me. I've already lived with a co-wife for almost three years. (Madame HS5, secretary, 39 years old, six children, Talladjé district)

A third factor leading to abortion can be conjugal crisis. During periods when the bonds of marriage are weakened, some women take revenge on their husbands through abortion. This appears to be the ultimate "weapon of the weak" available to a married woman in the face of a social order that dictates her conduct (Scott 1985). One woman, Madame RC, a 32-year-old housewife, told me at the beginning of her interview that her marriage was struggling. Married for nine years, with three children, she had just aborted a seven-week pregnancy after having had a violent fight with her husband, who she described as "a big alcoholic." Madame RC had attempted but failed to provoke an abortion during her third pregnancy to protest her husband's plan to remarry. Situations of this kind are rare, however; and more often women try to overcome common social constraints by having more rather than fewer children:

> After all, even if you get along badly with a man, there's no reason to take it out on your pregnancy. Then the child will be the source of your future joy. (Madame HI, 29 years old, two children, gas station attendant, Gaweye district)

In the cases detailed above, we can see the elements of resistance to a social order. According to Koster, abortions performed within a conjugal context in Yoruba society can be a sign of resistance to the husband's patrilineage: "Abortion by a married woman is frowned upon because she denies her husband's patrilineage a child already conceived" (2003: 11). Koster notes that abortion might serve as a kind of "alternative norm in some groups to solve the problem of unwanted pregnancy; so might preventing pregnancy with dangerous and ineffective drugs" (2003: 307).

Abortion, like contraception, can sometimes serve to hide adultery committed by a married woman. Because a pregnancy in the absence of a married woman's husband puts her in a compromising situation, she often chooses to get rid of it. When a woman who appears to be pregnant ceases to be pregnant, those around her suspect her of adultery.

ABORTION IN THE FACE OF SOCIAL CRITICISM

In Niger, abortion is condemned by society and religion, and it is a criminal act punishable by the penal code. To date, no law authorizing abortion exists, and there is no social movement seeking its decriminalization. Abortion is therefore only an option if recommended by doctors to save the mother's life, a position adhered to in official health structures (Moussa Abdallah 2002: 108). Nevertheless, I am not aware of any criminal cases brought against a woman who has had an abortion. Abortion, though prohibited by law, is tolerated provided it remains hidden. By contrast, the justice system has been uncompromising in pursuing cases of infanticide committed by single women (young girls and divorced or widowed women), leading to imposing prison terms.[5]

Abortion runs against social laws and principles, attracting criticism. For example, Madame IR, 32 years of age, experienced a terminated pregnancy

5. Editor's note: Given how difficult it can be to distinguish a late-term miscarriage from infanticide, it may be that some unmarried women charged with infanticide had simply suffered a miscarriage or stillbirth.

in the third month of her pregnancy. In the absence of her husband, her in-laws suspected her of having ended her pregnancy. Her sister-in-law FI said, "I'm sure IR didn't miscarry. She didn't want that child. I think a lot of things are being hidden." One of Madame IR's cousins thinks more or less the same thing: "What IR did is horrible. She didn't have any health problems. So I don't see how she could've lost her child."

Despite it being mentioned often, abortion remains hidden "behind the scenes" of social life, as Erving Goffman would put it.[6] Unquestionably, abortion is a particularly sensitive subject because, as François-André Isambert observes, it is "at the heart of a series of tensions around notions of life, the relationship between law and morals, sexual ethics, the status of women, the rationality of reproductive decisions, the role of the medical institution" (1982: 380). Drawing upon both historical and anthropological data, Luc Boltanski attempts to understand why abortion remains secretive in France despite having been legal for decades. He argues that abortion remains secretive because of the tension between it and the main principles of the social contract, which promotes demographic renewal (Boltanski [2004] 2013: 34). Perceived as a social evil, abortion is absent from direct references, whether these are images or objects. As a result, it is difficult to study it as a subject. Abortion and representations of abortion escape public attention because information on anything related to it falls into the realm of an accusation, of placing blame. Chantal Horellou-Lafarge captures the coercive dimension of social surveillance in France: "as control of the birth rate is essential to social reproduction, abortion has often been seen as a fundamental form of social deviance" (1982: 397).

For everyone, the social framework is a controlling factor in one's sexual and reproductive life. A married woman's entourage (her parents, in-laws, friends, neighbors) monitors any transformation of her body. The suspicion of abortion hovers over some married women in this situation. This close, but sometimes unsuspected, surveillance influences the behavior of many individuals. The law of silence is a matter of course in the event of a voluntary termination of pregnancy. Some women deny having had an abortion so as not to risk exposure because, as one nurse put it, "walls have ears everywhere, but they also have eyes." People's fear of talking about a deliberate termination of pregnancy is matched only by the extent of the social condemnation that will follow if discovered.

6. Editor's note: Interestingly, it seems that Goffman initially borrowed the image from Simone de Beauvoir (see Goffman 1959: 113).

The overwhelming majority of Nigeriens are Muslim. The dominant Islamic religious culture of Niger argues (as among many Christians) that neither an embryo nor a fetus should be suppressed because Islam prohibits ending a human life.[7] Important ethical considerations on the rights of a fetus as well as on the idea of the human have been put forward. This view of the termination of pregnancy rules it an infanticide:

> It's an abomination to kill a child, even if it's not yet born. You will answer to God since you want to change what He has decided. A human cannot end the life of another, even that of her child. (Alpha HO, 46 years old, marabout, Gaweye district)

This type of normative framing keeps individuals who have had an abortion in "guilty" silence. It applies to married women when they cannot convince others of the spontaneous and involuntary nature of the end of their pregnancy. This strong disapproval of abortion in most discourses is due to the perception that it results from irreligion and the disintegration of morals. It is no coincidence that a strong moral system surrounds abortion and its interpretation.

> Abortion is *haram* [sacrilege, taboo, contrary to religious rules]. Women are having more and more abortions because *ceferitarey* ([Z] paganism) is also very common.[8] People don't respect traditions or religion, so they break all the rules, do things as they please. (Alpha HI, 41 years old, marabout, Lamordé district)

The only exception to this rule, according to Malam AY, a member of the Society of Islamic Associations for Family Planning and Social Development (Groupement des Associations Islamiques en matière de Planification Familiale et Développement Sociale), is when a pregnancy is harmful to the life of the woman or that of her child: "A woman is allowed to have an abortion when her pregnancy can harm her or the baby she's carrying."

7. Editor's note: The permissibility of contraception and abortion is the subject of debate among scholars of Islam. It is possible to mount an Islamic rationale for both contraception and abortion in the context of marriage, but such positions are not common in Niger. HM assumes that all Christians see abortion as murder, which is inaccurate. Since many Christians she would have known in Niger are Catholic, we have changed "Christianity" to "among many Christians."

8. Editor's note: *Ceferi tarey* is derived from the Arabic word for "unbelief" (*kufr*), which by extension refers to non-Muslims. Implicitly no true Muslim would have an abortion.

This social and religious rigidity goes beyond Niger. Despite its legal nature in France, Boltanski tells us, there is still great difficulty in talking about abortion because the act is still subject to widespread social reprobation: "It is very rare that abortion is accepted in principle, including in societies where its practice is frequent . . . although we know that 'it exists', such a practice can concern neither relatives nor even the social group to which one belongs" (2004: 30). This can be observed in Africa. Koster has identified this attitude in some Yoruba women who have had abortions themselves: "Most women, even those who have had an abortion, disapprove of it and morally evaluate other women who did it, referring to the norms they themselves violated" (2003: 306).

LOCAL PHRASEOLOGY SURROUNDING ABORTION

In the Hausa and Zarma languages, the semantics vary depending on whether a woman has had a miscarriage or an abortion. In the case of miscarriage, a chain of solidarity and compassion is formed to support a grieving mother. Conversely, indignation and stigma meet those who have had an abortion.

A miscarriage generally gives rise to commiseration from friends, parents, and caregivers. Overall, everyone agrees that it was not deliberately caused by the woman who carried the pregnancy; any idea of intentionality is rejected. Here, something acts upon the female subject. As a result, a "natural" abortion is generally linked to illness. A woman's poor health may be seen as the cause of a miscarriage. Malaria and fever are the most cited pathologies. A spontaneous abortion is also attributable to the "evil eye" or to the "evil tongue," which signifies that the mother has been the victim of symbolic malice. Bad luck (*kotte* [Z] and *asiiri* or *magani* [H]) and witchcraft (*cerkawtaray* [Z] and *maita* [H]) can also cause a miscarriage. Finally, many people think that mystical forces or spirits (called *jinns*) can cause the disappearance of a pregnancy. Spontaneous abortion is a passive experience endured by a woman. In Hausa, it is called *barnan ciki* or *bari* and in Zarma *gunde hasaraw* or *gunde kan yan*. In both languages, this corresponds literally to "belly damage," "falling belly," or "fallen belly."

As the result of human compassion for her *hasaraw* ("loss" [Z]), a woman benefits from solidarity often in the form of visitors offering encouragement. All wishes or prayers expressed are that this lost fruit may be quickly replaced. These types of visits are similar to those made following a bereavement. In this situation, the woman is a victim who is pitied.

A woman who has lost a pregnancy is, in some ways, a grieving woman who is offered condolences. She needs support. She should be given hope for a new pregnancy and a happy ending. (Madame HB2, 47 years old, five children, companion of a woman giving birth, Talladjé Maternity Ward)

In the case of an abortion, the ideas of provocation and intentionality are captured in Zarma expressions such as *gunde zeeriyan* ("leveling the belly"), *gunde furu yan* ("throwing away the belly," "rejected belly"), *gunde dooru yan* ("disposing of the belly"), or *gunde mun yan* ("pouring out the belly"). The idea of "pouring out the belly" also exists in Hausa, where the phrase *zubda ciki* is used. In these contexts, words, phrases, and sentences tend to represent the premeditation of the action, as well as the social disapproval that is attached to it. Even a woman who faces life-threatening conditions as a result of a botched abortion receives little commiseration. Such a woman is considered a culprit who is to be blamed:

If you're capable of aborting, you're also capable of killing a person. Life is a sacred thing. When you think there are people who've never had children, it's an insult to see others take away lives. (Madame AS, 31 years old, four children, wife of a marabout, Talladjé district)

Ultimately, miscarriage and abortion are socially registered in a dichotomous view. From one side (spontaneous abortion) to the other (induced abortion) the woman is considered either a victim or a culprit.

ABORTIVE TECHNIQUES

Abortion medications and practices vary from one case to another. Due to the non-legal nature of these services, it was impossible for me to observe the use of these techniques directly. Regardless of the setting where women seek an abortion, secrecy is a primary objective.

Abortive Practices in the Popular Sphere

I was not able to specifically identify abortive substances recommended or practices done by Muslim healers or by traditional healers. That does not necessarily mean that marabouts and traditional healers do not provide "remedies" that are said to be abortive. Popular abortive processes seem to be more of a feminine therapeutic craft related to knowledge of how to cause the return of menstruation through emmenagogues. The choices regarding ingredients take into account the effects that these abortive methods can have on a pregnancy. It is therefore their proven noxious nature that draws a woman toward to them. They must also be applied in excess to ensure the operation's success. Harmful products must be consumed in large quantities. These ingredients are typically very sour, very sweet, very hot, very bitter, or very acidic. Certain drugs, such as Nivaquine and aspirin, are commonly used in attempts to induce abortion.

Breaking Behavioral Norms

Before turning to "dangerous products," a woman seeking to terminate her pregnancy will often try to defy the cultural prohibitions (behavioral and nutritional) for expecting women. Because popular representations mention the carrying of heavy weights as likely to cause a miscarriage, some women go out of their way to perform such labor. Women are also told quite vehemently to avoid certain movements, practices, and positions during pregnancy; women who want to have an abortion reverse these recommendations. Because strong pressure on the stomach is discouraged, the stomach may be tied tightly with a loincloth, which is often supported by a thin rope. Some women attempt dangerous movements that can cause falls and consequently trigger a miscarriage.

Further, millet stalks are often used as probes inserted into the vagina. This is one of the most dangerous methods of abortion since the stems can cause hemorrhaging, infections, and quite often tetanus.

Finally, there are prohibitions on bloodletting for pregnant women. Bloodletting is a common traditional practice in the humoral tradition that is performed by a traditional barber called a *wanzami* (H), who also performs circumcisions of boys, uvulectomy, and scarification. This practice is disappearing with the discouragement of cutting due to both the danger of tetanus and the possible transmission of HIV. The *wanzami* drains some blood from the woman, who is fully aware of the possible side effects that it can cause, such as loss of the embryo or fetus. Bloodletting can often turn into severe bleeding. Some women practice bloodletting themselves.

Defying Dietary Restrictions

A woman may attempt to disrupt a pregnancy by defying the many nutritional taboos imposed upon pregnant women. Among the foods prohibited for pregnant women are those that are too sweet, too hot, too salty, and too spicy.

Taking "Dangerous" Products

If the above-mentioned approaches fail, more aggressive methods may be used. This includes turning to products and techniques known to be harmful to pregnant women to induce an abortion. Some of the same products are used as contraceptives. Various antiseptic products are included in the repertoire of abortive products used locally. According to some respondents, purges and vaginal or rectal enemas can also be carried out using certain "dangerous products" to provoke an abortion.

Similar to bleach and used for its disinfecting properties, potassium permanganate is thought to cause perforations inside the uterus. It is believed that this caustic product, when diluted, can be ingested. It is also said to be very dangerous; an overdose can cause death. Ginger and chili, designated as aphrodisiacs, are both used for their supposed toxicity. These products, transformed into powder, are macerated in water and then consumed together or separately. Patients who mix them are generally in a hurry for immediate results. In either case, the ingested product, which overheats the stomach because of its tonic quality, facilitates purging or enema. The enema can also be inserted rectally.

Azadirachta indica, or neem, is a common plant whose seeds are often transformed into oil for use in soap making.[9] It is a very corrosive plant and therefore has abortive properties that are highly sought after. Both its leaves and seeds, even when used separately, are believed to be effective for carrying out an abortion. Senegal mahogany, *Khaya senegalensis*, is a particularly bitter plant known as *madacci* (H) or *farre* (Z) locally. Traditional healers prescribe it to fight dysentery (*woyno* [Z] or *zahi* [H]). Women who use this product most often do so claiming to suffer from *woyno*, a local disease category that is vague and common in Niger (Olivier de Sardan 1999b). Women may also use suppositories (referred to as "*ovules*" [Fr. eggs]) that consist of a mixture of plants with abortive properties that are transformed into powder, then kneaded into a dough. This mixture, often accompanied by a lubricant, is introduced into the vagina, against the cervix, for a period varying from half an hour to two hours.

9. Also called Indian lilac, neem is designated by the words *beedi* or *dogon yaaro* (H) and *miliyâ* (Z) (Bernard and White-Kaba 1994: 227).

Because sweetness is dangerous, sugar is seen as a substance that facilitates abortion; products are often taken together with Coca-Cola, which is also favored for its effervescence. Women may also use a vaginal tampon or cotton soaked in lemon, vinegar, bleach, or permanganate.

Without giving an exact description of how they are used, saffron, soap, and henna (also used as a contraceptive) are included in the repertoire of abortive products used locally. Some respondents had experienced the dangers of toxicity in their own families:

> One of my relatives died after consuming a henna solution. People had told her that this product would give her an abortion. She was able to have the abortion, but she died soon after. She had abdominal pain for almost three days and eventually died.

The Use of Pharmaceuticals

Abortive properties are also attributed to pharmaceutical products that are contraindicated for use during pregnancy. On this subject, Koster remarks that among Yoruba women in Nigeria, "If rumors are spread that a certain drug should not be used during pregnancy, girls and women want to believe it can abort their unwanted pregnancy" (2003: 301). For example, Nivaquine is used as a cure or prophylactic for malaria.[10] Among young adolescents, it is known to have deadly properties. Another commonly available drug, effervescent aspirin (or Efferalgan), is taken in overdose with the hope that it will produce the same effects as Nivaquine. Most suicide attempts involve an overdose of Nivaquine. By extension, it is often understood to suppress an unwanted pregnancy.

> It is generally believed that one can get rid of an early pregnancy (less than three months) by taking between eight and 12 Nivaquine tablets. Nivaquine is a very easily accessible drug. You don't need a prescription for it, nor is it necessary to go to a health center to get it. It's sold in pharmacies without any questions, and street vendors bring it to your door to ensure total discretion. It's the lack of constraints and prohibitions around this drug that makes it popular among women wishing to have a secret abortion. Moreover, for young girls it's the first, if not the main, remedy. (Midwife, Niamey, CNSR)

10. Editor's note: Nivaquine, the most commonly used antimalarial agent in Niger and Nigeria, is composed of the alkaloid sulfate salt chloroquine sulfate.

Madame HI, a 26-year-old married woman whose husband has been absent for 11 months, is suspected by her sister-in-law of having taken a large dose of Nivaquine in order to have an abortion:

> I saw my sister-in-law take seven Nivaquine tablets at the same time. Faced with my surprise, she told me she wanted to give herself a shock treatment for malaria. Fifteen minutes later, my little sister, who lives in her house, told me that she'd caught HI taking a large number of tablets. That day, she was hospitalized with the help of her nurse friend. She arranged things so the family couldn't visit her for two days on medical grounds. Personally, I'd suspected she was pregnant, but a week later when she was discharged from the hospital, all signs of pregnancy had disappeared. . . . My brother, who suspected her of not being faithful, repudiated her on his return. (Madame RB, 35 years old, six children, shopkeeper, Gaweye district)

Various kinds of capsules commonly called *tupay* (or *toupaille*) feature among remedies sought for an abortion.[11] According to Laurent Chilliot (2003: 456), "Tupay is the name given to two-color tetracycline capsules whose uses are extremely diverse. . . . Yet today, this term tends to encompass all pill capsules (mostly antibiotics, given their diversity on the informal market)." The composition of these drugs is varied: antibiotics (such as ampicillin or tetracycline), anti-diarrheal drugs, analgesics, anti-depressants, or vitamins (Moussa Abdallah 2001). I did not find any *tupay* with exclusively abortive properties. As with other kinds of tablets, women seeking abortions rely primarily on the effects of overdose to bring an end to an unwanted pregnancy.

Abortion Cocktails

Women also make use of abortive "cocktails" made from different pharmaceutical products in various combinations. Nivaquine–tupay, effervescent aspirin–tupay, and Nivaquine–pill, among others, are cited as being abortive cocktails.

---

11. The transcription varies according to different authors: *toupaille* (Haxaire 2003) and *tupay* (Chilliot 2003). Editor's note: Chilliot explores *tupay* in the context of local understandings of infectious disease transmission. Interestingly, Haxaire shows that *toupaille* are also understood to be a remedy for infertility since they can cure sexually transmitted infections.

In addition, those considering abortion employ what Gélis (1984) calls "the 'sympathy' of color." Red is usually the color of choice. For these women, it is a question of "turning to the color red in order, of course, to see 'red.'" This corresponds to what Gélis calls a "pharmacopoeia of analogy." In Niamey, for example, some women use palm or beetroot oil for their red color. I could not obtain directions for the use of these products.

Many other abortive methods were identified, some being founded upon heat, which is supposed to contribute to the blood's liquefaction. Thus, drinking boiling beverages, sitting on the place where the oven sat while cooking the meal, or being exposed to the sun for long periods are all part of the "hot" abortive methods. One of my interviewees offered this story about a high school student:

> One of my husband's nieces drank boiling tapioca to the point of burning her tongue and gums. Two days earlier, she'd heard that high heat can cause an abortion. It killed her—she complained of excruciating pain in her stomach, throat, and mouth. She also bled for two days. The first day, the family didn't know. The second day when we found out, we took her to the hospital. There, we were told that it was a case for the maternity ward. But it was too late; she died from a hemorrhage due to excessive heat. That was when we learned that she'd tried to abort. It was also at that moment that her mother learned she was pregnant. (Madame GH, 55 years old, four children, companion of a woman giving birth, Gaweye district)

All these methods are self-administered. Because of the proprietary and sometimes occult nature of these "remedies," I was not able to learn much about how these substances were actually used by healers and marabouts. Furthermore, I was unable to establish the presence of "angel makers"—women who make a profession of providing illegal abortion services. Such women exist in other sociocultural settings, but I was unable to identify or interview any in Niger.[12]

Medical and Surgical Abortive Practices

The anti-gestation and anti-progestin drugs mifepristone (also called RU-486) and misoprostol have not yet been tested for use by the Nigerien

12. Editor's note: French law and literature of the 19th century used the expression *faiseuse d'ange* (angel maker) to refer to what in English would be a "back-alley abortionist." The French term assumes all abortionists are women.

medical community.[13] Women who approach public medical structures for illicit or health-related abortion are generally limited to curettage treatments.[14] Therefore, although the methods presented below draw upon biomedical pharmacology products, they are not always dispensed by healthcare professionals; and if they are, they are not always accessible to the public. According to my research, the most common methods used in the medical environment are injections of oxytocin to induce labor, curettage, and probes.

Synthocinon (oxytocin), commonly known as "syntho," is readily available in Niger because it is administered intravenously to promote contractions during delivery in clinical settings. Even when it is not necessary, nursing staff may administer it to women in labor to charge money that they then pocket. This product is increasingly used for purposes other than its primary therapeutic objective, namely abortion (Souley 2003; Moussa 2004b). Because its administration requires a minimum of medical knowledge, "syntho" is commonly cited as an abortive remedy employed in the biomedical sphere. One civil servant recounted how she had an abortion in a public health center:

> Thanks to help from a school friend, I was put on syntho for a day at the dispensary in. . . . They gave me an injection first . . . . At the end of the day, I bled heavily. That was how I lost my six-week pregnancy. (Madame KR, 33 years old, four children, Balafon district)

Dilation and curettage entails the dilation of the cervix, followed by the scraping of the uterine wall with a curette to empty it of its contents; it requires medical expertise, and therefore, according to many of my respondents, it is only performed by healthcare specialists. Some women made reference to "abortion specialists," presumably medical staff, who

13. Editor's note: A "medical" or medication abortion is a procedure that uses medication to end a pregnancy. It requires no surgery or anesthesia. An "in-clinic" or "surgical" abortion might involve vacuum aspiration or dilation and evacuation and must be carried out by a trained medical specialist. According to Guillaume (2009: 8), the distribution of RU-486 across Africa has only started in South Africa and Tunisia where abortion is legal.

14. Editor's note: At the time of HM's research the situation was shifting as a result of international pressure upon governments to provide post-abortion care to women, regardless of the legal status of abortion. As a result, some specialists in Niger have been trained in how to use the post-abortion package of care including vacuum aspiration and the drug misprostol. Mifepristone is also available in a form intended to treat hyperglycemia (Korlym) in Niger. Inevitably, stocks make their way to the black market. Nevertheless, attitudes of nurses and midwives toward abortion are very negative, particularly if it concerns an unmarried woman (Diarra et al. 2017).

"introduced a hand into the uterus" to remove the embryo or fetus. They may have been referring to manual vacuum aspiration using a special syringe to apply suction.

Beyond these biomedical abortive procedures available illicitly in Niamey, some women seek treatment internationally. They travel to neighboring countries to end an unwanted pregnancy far from suspicious eyes and networks of acquaintances. Many women from Niamey and its periphery, as well as those living in the interior of the country, are said to travel to border countries such as Nigeria, Burkina Faso, and Benin. These destinations serve women in search of "guaranteed"—and above all discreet—abortion methods. For women in Niamey, the most common path is to Benin, particularly the city of Malanville. Abou-Bakari Imorou identified civil servants from the Beninese public sector (in particular from the hospital) with private practices in Malanville who "are for the most part renowned practitioners of abortions and whose clientele is largely Nigerien" (2006: 318). Surveillance and prosecution for abortion were more prevalent under the Kountché regime than they are today under a democratic regime. Imorou observes that the Nigerien clientele were more numerous during Kountché's time in power. He suggests that these kinds of specialized private practice reveal that "there is a significant demand which is not taken into account by public care services—at least not formally" (2006: 318). Cities like Malanville have thus become a refuge for abortion specialists, who are found there in not insignificant numbers and offer a broad range of methods beyond those available in Niamey.

CONCLUSION

Women make use of contraception and abortion as tools in a struggle to master their own maternal destiny. While they may have little control over their sexuality, they nevertheless can take action to prevent having a child. Contraception, depending upon the form it takes, may require women to maneuver complex and constraining terrain. Women may attempt to negotiate to open up their options within their conjugal context, outside the household, with their kin, and in health centers. But they do not always succeed, and when they don't they may draw upon a more "extreme" (in their words) mode of contraception, namely abortion. The use of "contraception" abortion reveals the depth and power of contradictory social injunctions upon married women.

Conclusion: Fertility Management in Niger

This study of the management of fertility in Niger seeks to attract attention to an issue that is still under-investigated in the social sciences. In this analysis of infertile sexuality, I have conceptualized infertility as both the impossibility of conceiving and the refusal of childbearing (Gélis 1984). These two forms of infertile sexuality reveal how a society regulates fertility in various ways. At both the macroscopic and the microscopic levels, society asserts control over fertility at every stage. Through geographic proximity and kinship ties, relatives, friends, acquaintances, allies, and even neighbors intrude into the life of the household. In general, these social interventions promote natalism. The experience of pervasive social surveillance can hinder the construction of an autonomous self. Both individuals and society as a whole are captive to this dynamic (Donati 2000). These forces at multiple scales—produced by the marital unit, relatives, the medical system, and popular care networks—create a multitude of norms, some convergent, others contradictory.

Several conclusions can be drawn from this study. First, individual decision-making confronts a plurality of social and moral norms, each of which is interwoven with multiple social practices. Second, in the social spheres I have studied (e.g., the matrimonial home and family, the broader popular sphere, the biomedical sphere), fertility regulation, especially for women, entails direct and indirect interventions on the body. The collective management of human reproduction involves the multifaceted control of women's bodies. Finally, women, though they face numerous constraints, are not passive. They deploy a variety of microstrategies that give evidence of their ambivalence toward the social order.

Concerns related to fertility and its management permeate the experience of individuals in every aspect of life—social, economic, political, symbolic, and religious—constituting the quintessential "total social phenomenon" explored by Marcel Mauss in his study, *The Gift*: "In these total social phenomena, as we propose to call them, all kinds of institutions find simultaneous expression: religious, legal, moral, and economic" (1954: 1).[1]

A MULTITUDE OF STANDARDS

The cult of natalism combined with stigmatization of closely spaced births means that most people are faced with contradictory injunctions, or a double-bind. Gregory Bateson, in the context of "schizophrenic communication," explains:

> From the point of view of the patient, the contexts have the following formal structure: a parent whom he intensely both loves and hates emits signals of an incongruent nature. This incongruence is perhaps most clear when one half of the parent's behavior precedes an act of the patient and the other half follows. The parent will, for example, incite the patient to express a courageous opinion, and when that opinion is expressed, will disparage it as unloving, disloyal, disobedient, etc. Characteristically, the first half of the parent's behavior will appear to be set in a certain mode or philosophy of interpersonal relations, while the second half is a denial of this mode and the substitution of another. (1991: 116)[2]

There is therefore a flagrant contradiction between the celebration of motherhood and the condemnation of *nasu* (Z) or *rusutsa* ([H] close pregnancies). In-laws are particularly notorious for enforcing these types of conflicting or even "capricious" logics (*fundi baayi* [Z]), as this respondent points out:

1. Editor's note: We have inserted this key passage from Marcel Mauss' *The Gift*, which HM assumes the reader will know well. This concluding reference to *The Gift* is important because the obligation to produce children to make good on the conjugal debt is exactly the kind of seemingly disinterested and voluntary transaction that Mauss shows is in fact obligatory and bound up in questions of social hierarchy, property, and belonging.
2. Editor's note: HM assumes the reader will already be familiar with the "double bind" theory. We have inserted this passage from Bateson (1991) to flesh out HM's reference and to emphasize that the theory has relevance for the psychological experience of the patient, who is in this instance diagnosed with schizophrenia. The double bind is form of psychic violence that not all are able to surmount.

When you give birth to a lot of children, they never leave you alone; if you don't give birth to any, you never have peace. If you don't give birth, they'll say to their son, "You've married a *gabdi* that you're feeding without children. Divorce her and look for another wife." If they hate you, you'll have no respite. (Madame MY, 52 years old, nine children, Gaweye neighborhood)

Researchers are often confronted with what appear to be inconsistencies when talking with informants, who express differing rhetoric depending upon the circumstances and interests that are at stake. As Luc Boltanski notes,

> moral sociology does not necessarily require that all moral references on the part of actors be taken at face value, but it does require at the very least that sociologists take such references seriously, in order to study the way actors themselves deal with the gap between normative requirements and reality, whether by critiquing the world as it is or, on the contrary, by justifying themselves in response to critiques ([2004] 2013: 4)

The researcher encounters these gaps between the normative and the reality particularly frequently when addressing issues related to gender. In part, this is because sexual categorizations are variable and malleable and shift from one social field to another even within a single milieu (Daune-Richard and Hurtig 1995).

In this mountain of conflicting expectations and standards, those transmitted through religion dominate decisively. Some conservative religious leaders preach incessantly on issues related to human reproduction and to social relations between men and women. In general, religion socializes the individual by "taming" freedom of thought. In Niamey, most Islamic education directed toward Muslim women—which is closely linked to an urban religious style—elaborates arguments for imposing the rigor of a bygone era upon women. Islamic rules are applied to excess by fanatic groups upon Muslim women. According to Bouhdiba (2001), the lack of consensus over Islamic norms results to some degree from ambiguities and contradictions in Islamic texts.

Yet wherever people face a multitude of social, religious, and moral prescriptions out of synch with reality, individuals fashion their own "practical norms" that are, in a way, a form of insubordination, however modest (Olivier de Sardan 2001b). This is especially characteristic of women, who rarely rebel openly and directly. They use what Scott (1985) calls the "weapons of the weak" to mount subtle combat against an ideology or value system.

Because "self-ownership" begins with that of the body (Fraisse 1998), the appropriation or reappropriation of women's own bodies is a prerequisite for their emancipation. In addition to being our immediate reference for human identity, the body is a marker of otherness linked to individuality (Le Breton 2003). This otherness, however, is often subject to certain forms of violation. Of all the forms of domestication of the female body, control over sexuality appears to be the most palpable and the most successful. Thus, the inviolability of the conjugal debt, which is institutionalized in Islam, serves as a pretext and foundation for the perpetuation of male domination. The conjugal debt is indeed one of the strongest indicators of sexual hierarchy in a society. Theoretically applicable to both spouses, marital duty has, in fact, been enforced solely for the benefit of men.

The female body meets a triple societal need: it is a sexual object, a reproductive machine, and an aesthetic object that often serves the purpose of ensuring male prestige (Tabet 1998; Knibiehler 2001; Mathieu 1985). It follows from the differentiation of the sexes that the female body is appropriated more frequently than the male body. Marie Hélène Mottin Sylla (1997) observes that in Africa the praise given to the fertility of women goes hand in hand with an appropriation of women's bodies by society, which is regulated by the male "mass." Free choice in sexuality and fertility cannot be given free expression in women. While the radicalism of some of these authors calls for some tempering, it is clear that the body serves as one important interface in the domination of women. In general, in addition to the feminization of conjugal debt, the refusal to allow or the imposition of contraceptive use on women, the practice of excision, forced or subtle sterilization of girls or women, son preference and sex-selective abortion, and rape are all palpable indicators of different forms of appropriation and domestication of the female body by men. This book has shed light on the first two, proving, if need be, that the woman's body is under control.

The gradual disjunction between procreation and pleasure elsewhere, due to various sociocultural changes, has not yet prompted unconstrained sexuality in Niger. Invisible barriers (standards and prejudices underlying gender relations) still exist, and the traditional order, fueled by religious extremism, is still very much present in women's daily lives. In Niger, power relations are most often played out to the detriment of women. Conceptions of and behaviors related to fertility are difficult to change; the individual and collective internalization of the dominant modes of thought guarantees their perpetuation (Ryckmans 1997).

In Niamey, women do not have a personal maternal project as envisioned in the contemporary West so much as a socially mandated maternal destiny. The family circle will defend this pro-natal reproductive norm fiercely. The pro-natalist leitmotif revealed in interviews confirmed that in Niger, as in medieval Europe, "sexual morality necessarily leads to a pro-life philosophy" (Bologne 1988: 276). Further, the same sexual morality in some "advanced" countries has meant that the right to abortion and access to contraception are very recent, and individuals continue to face significant practical constraints (Boltanski [2004] 2013). Fertility management in Niger almost universally implies the rejection of contraception, particularly in its modern form, by husbands and their families, resulting in a low contraceptive prevalence rate.

The regulation of a couple's fertility is justified in the name of the protection of the family lineage. This requires monitoring and control over female sexuality to produce an unequivocally "clean birth" (Lacoste-Dujardin [1985] 1996). Moreover, a woman who has not reserved sexual "primary exclusivity" for her husband at the time of her first marriage is more exposed to this surveillance and to all kinds of suspicious suppositions (Goffman 1977). Communal ontological necessity—which is itself part of a process of social domination—is invoked to control women. This control, to be effective and sustainable, also employs a multitude of moral and religious constraints that I have described in this book. Often, women support this ideology themselves. The perpetuation of male domination would not be possible without the conscious or unconscious actions of other women.

REGULATING FERTILITY IN MEDICAL HEALTH CENTERS: A HIGHLY ADVOCATED CONTRACEPTIVE STANDARD

The potential to make use of contraception generates power relations between healthcare providers and users (patients and, to some extent, their husbands and families) within health centers. Observation of interactions between caregivers and clients has enabled me to recognize how the progressive medicalization of the human body in general, and of women in particular, is effectively a form of control over individuals. The ideal promoted in medical settings is a "contraceptive standard" through which women are expected to adhere to norms linked to biomedical contraceptive technologies. As a result, the female body is increasingly part of an institutional control system that promotes the governing of the body (Fassin and Memmi 2004; Foucault 1986). In health facilities contraceptive practice also occasions the manipulation of women's bodies (e.g., through the insertion of an intrauterine device, the implantation of Norplant). This is evidenced in the often cavalier and routine way in which contraceptives are prescribed to patients coming to postpartum consultations. Thus, in addition to the treatment of infertility and the management of pregnancies and childbirth—which require manipulation and direct physical intervention—the medical system is again invited to manage bodies in the provision of contraception. This management materializes in the form of a "disappropriation" of the body (Locoh and Sztalryd 1995).

My research has found that many women accept in principle the idea of contraception, including the use of biomedical contraceptive medicine. I argued that if the use of medical contraception is less successful than it might be, one main reason is that, unlike the provision of healthcare in other social spaces in Niamey, medical centers are culturally unwelcoming spaces for most women. Unless patients are of the same social status as the clinic personnel, they are treated as inferior. A strong social hierarchy is experienced negatively by ordinary women during family planning consultations. Inconsiderate health staff, interminably long wait times, and violations of patient–provider privacy are among the many sources of frustration for clients. At the same time, healthcare providers complain of "bad patients" who fail to follow instructions or to come to appointments. These tense social relationships pose a significant barrier to the use of medical contraception.

REGULATING FERTILITY IN THE POPULAR HEALTH SPHERE: HYBRID NORMS

In the popular realm of healthcare, women reveal their own complex desires to both produce children and control the timing or deferral of pregnancies. For some women, the reproductive norm and the contraceptive standard converge and become indistinguishable—contraception accords with the goal of numerous, well-spaced children. Women's choices are therefore pragmatic: they may adhere to hybrid or heterogeneous standards, resulting at times in normative and therapeutic syncretism. While traditional healers and marabouts use their therapies to help women manage pregnancies, space births, or combat infertility, street vendors offer them contraceptives, stimulants, and abortive products.

The traditional healers' and marabouts' therapeutic actions are directed almost exclusively at the female body through concoctions, fumigations, medications, invocations, rituals of possession, bleeding, and physical interventions on genitalia. Infertile women, in their therapeutic quest, undergo or inflict upon themselves a form of dispossession of their bodies. Fertile women as well negotiate between reproductive and contraceptive norms. They approach the popular therapeutic sphere (as opposed to biomedical spaces) to secure a pregnancy and to ensure their own health during this crucial period of their lives. There is always a fear that pregnancy might prove fatal. Marabouts and healers, more than the biomedical community, are there to reassure women.

Ultimately, the study of the multifaceted management of fertility involves observing gender relationships in a family setting, difficult and conflictual interactions in health centers, and the wider and more easily negotiable specialized popular health sphere.

NO CHILD, NO SOCIAL EXISTENCE

One of the main consequences of the absence of children in a woman's life is a far-reaching "social absence," which deeply affects her. Female identity in Niger entails successful reproduction. All symbolism of femininity revolves around motherhood. This conditions a woman experiencing infertility to undertake a conscious or unconscious "self-effacement" or to fall into a hypersensitive self-hatred psychoanalysts call "collapsed narcissism." Infertility feeds what Bessoles (2001) terms "lineage malaise" because the woman who remains beholden to the debt of life also puts herself in the position of one who will never be an ancestor. Social mobilization to protect and celebrate a woman who gives birth is far more sustained than that directed toward a woman in search of a child. As a result, infertile people, while suffering from discriminatory treatment, also receive little material and psychological support. Although not entirely alone, the childless woman has little companionship in her therapeutic quest. The "outsider" status that she occupies as an in-law in her husband's family further emphasizes her sense of isolation and social invisibility.

FEMALE FERTILITY MANAGEMENT AND THE KALEIDOSCOPE OF EMOTIONS

The study of fertility brings into relief many kinds of emotions. The expression of these feelings becomes all the more perceptible when the birth of a child is compromised or permanently delayed. A source of major anxiety, infertility upsets and weakens the status of women in the home but also in society. Whereas childbearing confers power, the infertile woman's body creates a rupture in the transmission of norms, values, practices, and achievements of all kinds. Psychologically and emotionally, women are affected, unconsciously internalizing a set of beliefs and representations that often frame infertile women as the culprit.

In this book, I have noted that women experiencing infertility often have contradictory feelings. A host of affective dispositions—love, brooding, shame, guilt, loneliness, anxiety, hope, and despair—punctuate the daily life of many of the childless women I met. Many childless women seem to have succumbed to a life of victimhood (Cyrulnik 2000) where they castigate themselves more than they are stigmatized by others. Guilt-laden rhetoric is met by an equally weighty rhetoric of victimization. Infertility poses one of the most profound crises for couples, which also affects the relationships of women to those around them (parents, friends, acquaintances, neighbors) and to their dreams for the future. Ultimately, many childless women close themselves off from others.

A holistic study of the emotions of women struggling with infertility captures the complexity of the human experience in ways that a narrow disciplinary approach cannot. Private life is the primary sanctuary of the emotional experience. In exploring the depths of human sensibilities, anthropology complements psychology while enriching its own analysis. Anthropology seeks not to erase these sentiments but rather to enhance our understanding of their significance (e.g., in the context of a therapeutic relationship in a healthcare setting, see Jaffré 2003d).

FROM WOMEN'S MICROSTRATEGIES TO "SILENT" REVOLT

In the face of multiple contradictory constraints, women do not necessarily sink into passivity. They sometimes deploy microstrategies that reveal their own preferences despite the social order. They use "women's tricks" to mount subtle combat against a restrictive ideology or value system. Within the dominant environment, the social actor deploys adaptive "tactics" (de Certeau 1990).

How do women "resist" the tyranny of social norms? The refusal of the conjugal debt, the deployment (or the rejection) of contraception, abortion, and adultery are among the many tactics that I have identified in this book. Depending on their circumstances, women sometimes quite creatively deny men their socially institutionalized sexual privileges. In opposition to the preferences of their spouses or family members, many women in Niamey impose spacing or even limitation of births by using biomedical contraceptives. Some women counter pro-natal social prescriptions through one or more abortions. Moreover, paradoxically, some women reject the family planning measures imposed by their spouses. Where men may take advantage of polygamy to counter sterility in a conjugal pairing, "infertile" women sometimes test their own reproductive capacities through adultery.

Apart from going on a sex strike, women almost always take roundabout and secretive measures to escape the hold of men, social rules, and religious prescriptions. The tactics most often used to circumvent and "fight" the power and domination of men do not challenge the status quo. Women have ways of subverting the social order, but it is often done so quietly, in ways that are not visible in the public sphere. When it comes to medical contraception and evading the conjugal debt, the exercise of women's agency happens at the margins.

CONCLUSION

In this study, I have combined approaches from symbolic anthropology (to grasp broad social understandings of fertility and infertility, kinship, filial ties, and matrimonial regimes), the anthropology of affect (to understand individuals' emotional universes), the sociology of decision-making (to examine an actor's rationality), and interactionist sociology (to analyze the construction of self and meaning through social interactions). My goal has been to capture the heterogeneity of experiences, emotions, and expectations that women, like any "plural actor," encounter and deploy depending on the circumstance (Lahire 1998).

At the very moment that Salafist Islamism is growing, we have seen the development and adoption of national and international legal instruments that contribute to the empowerment of women. We will therefore witness continuing confrontation and negotiation between spouses, between relatives and spouses, between the state and religious institutions, and between the state and its international financial and economic partners. My work here has taken up the central question of gender relations at the interstices of the conjugal cell and the kinship network. Much work remains to be done in tracing the development of contests and debates over gender relations in global and national public spaces.

BIBLIOGRAPHY

Adam, Michel. 1994. La femme Africaine: mère nourricière ou mère dévorante. Paper presented at the Congrès Afro-Brésilien IV Recife, Brazil, 17–20 April.

Alidou, Ousseina. 2005. *Engaging modernity: Muslim women and the politics of agency in postcolonial Niger*. Madison: University of Wisconsin Press.

Alio, Amina P., Laura Merrell, Kimberlee Roxburgh, et al. 2011. The psychosocial impact of vesico-vaginal fistula in Niger. *Archives of Gynecology and Obstetrics* 284: 371–378.

André, Jacques. 1985. Le coq et la jarre. *L'Homme* 25 (96): 49–75.

Andro, Armelle. 2001. Coopération et conflits entre conjoints en matière de reproduction en Afrique de l'Ouest. Thèse de doctorat de démographie, Université Paris X Nanterre.

Andro, Armelle, and Véronique Hertrich. 2001. La demande contraceptive au Sahel: les attentes des hommes se rapprochent-elles de celles de leurs épouses? *Population* 5: 721–770.

Attama, Sabine, Michka Seroussi, Alchina Idriss Kourguéni, et al. 1998. *Enquête démographique et de santé, Niger*. Calverton, MD: Care International/Niger and Macro International Inc.

Bajos, Nathalie, and Michèle Ferrand. 2004. La contraception, levier ou symbolique de la domination masculine? *Sciences sociales et santé* 22 (3): 117–140.

Bateson, Gregory. 1991. *A sacred unity: further steps to an ecology of mind*. San Francisco: HarperCollins.

Beauvoir, Simone de. 1973. *The second sex*. New York: Vintage Books.

Bernard, Yves, and Mary White-Kaba. 1994. *Dictionnaire Zarma-Français (République du Niger)*. Niamey: Agence de Coopération Culturelle et Technique.

Bessoles, Philippe. 2001. Infécondité féminine: un malaise dans la filiation. *Cliniques méditerranéennes* 63: 103–115.

Boerma, Jan Ties, and Zaida Mgalla. 2001. Introduction. In *Women and infertility in sub-Saharan Africa: a multidisciplinary perspective*, eds. Jan Ties Boerma and Zaida Mgalla, 13–24. Amsterdam: Kit Publishers.

Bologne, Jean-Claude. 1988. *La naissance interdite. Stérilité, avortement, contraception au moyen âge*. Paris: Éditions Olivier Orban.

Boltanski, Luc. 2004. *La condition fœtale: une sociologie de l'engendrement et de l'avortement*. Paris: Éditions Gallimard.

Bonnet, Doris. 1988. *Corps biologique, corps social. Procréation et maladies de l'enfant en pays mossi. Burkina Faso*. Paris: Éditions de l'ORSTOM.

Bonnet, Doris, and Agnès Guillaume. 1999. *La santé de la reproduction: concept et acteurs*. Documents de recherche 8. Paris: IRD.

Bouchard, Gérard. 2000. La sexualité comme pratique et rapport social chez les couples paysans du Saguenay (1860–1930). *Revue d'histoire de l'Amérique française* 54 (2): 183–217.

Bouhdiba, Abdelwahab. 2001. *La sexualité en Islam*. Paris: Presses universitaires de France.

Bozon, Michel. 1995. Les rapports entre femmes et hommes à la lumière des grandes enquêtes quantitatives. In *La place des femmes: Les enjeux de l'identité et de l'égalité au regard des sciences sociales*, ed. EPHESIA, 655–668. Paris: La Découverte.

Bozon, Michel. 2001. Sexualité et genre. In *Masculin–féminin: questions pour les sciences de l'homme*, eds. Jacqueline Laufer, Catherine Marry, and Margaret Maruani, 169–186. Paris: Presses universitaires de France.

Browner, Carole H., and Carolyn F. Sargent. 1996. The anthropology of human reproduction. In *Medical anthropology: contemporary theory and method*, eds. Carolyn F. Sargent and Thomas M. Johnson, 219–234. Westport, CT: Praeger.

Bureau Central du Recensement. 2004. *Résultats définitifs: répartition par sexe et par groupe d'âges de la population du Niger en 2001*. Niamey: Imprimerie NTI.

Bureau Central du Recensement. 2005. *Note de présentation des résultats définitifs, RGP/H-2001*. Niamey, Imprimerie NTI.

Bydlowski, Monique. 1997. *La dette de vie. Itinéraire psychanalytique de la maternité*. Paris: Presses universitaires de France.

Caldwell, John. 1982. *Theory of fertility decline*. London and New York: Academic Press.

Caldwell, John, and Patricia Caldwell. 1987. The cultural context of high fertility in sub-Saharan Africa. *Population and Development Review* 13 (3): 409–443.

CERPOD. 1996. *Santé de la reproduction au Sahel. Les jeunes en danger. Résultats d'une étude régionale dans cinq pays de l'Afrique de l'Ouest*. Dakar: CERPOD.

Chebel, Malek. 1984. *Le corps en Islam*. Paris: Presses Universitaires de France.

Chilliot, Laurent. 2003. Médicaments et prévention en milieu populaire Songhay-Zarma. In *Les maladies de passage. Transmissions, préventions et hygiènes en Afrique de l'Ouest*, eds. Doris Bonnet and Yanick Jaffré, 427–464. Paris: Karthala.

Coenen-Huther, Jacques. 1989. Parsons et Gurvitch: exigence de totalité et réciprocité de perspectives. *Sociologie et sociétés* XXI (1): 87–96.

Corbin, Alain. 1991. *Le temps, le desir et l'horreur: essais sur le dix-neuvième siècle*. Paris: Aubier-Montaigne.

Cosnier, Jacques. 1993. Les interactions en milieu soignant. In *Soins et communication. Approche interactionniste des relations de soins*, eds. Jacques Cosnier, Michèle Grosjean, and Michèle Lacoste, 17–32. Lyon: Presses universitaires de Lyon.

Cyrulnik, Boris. 2000. *Les nourritures affectives*. Paris: Éditions Odile Jacob.

Daune-Richard, Anne-Marie, and Marie-Claude Hurtig. 1995. Un débat loin d'être clos. In *La place des femmes. Les enjeux de l'identité et de l'égalité au regard des sciences sociales*, ed. EPHESIA, 426–438. Paris: La Découverte.

De Certeau, Michel. 1990. *L'invention du quotidien. Arts de faire*. Paris: Gallimard.

De Gaulejac, Vincent. 1996. *Les sources de la honte*. Paris: Desclée de Brouwer.

Delaisi de Parseval, Genevieve, and Alain Janaud. 1983. *L'enfant à tout prix*. Paris: Le Seuil.

Deutsch, Helène. [1949] 1987. *La psychologie des femmes. Maternité.* Vol. 2. Paris: Presses universitaires de France.

Devereux, George. 1955. *A study of abortion in primitive societies.* New York: The Julian Press.

Diarra, Aïssa, et al. 2017. Les interruptions volontaires de grossesse au Niger. *Études et travaux du LASDEL* 128: 1–88.

Diarra, Fatoumata Agnès. 1971. *Femmes Africaines en devenir. Les femmes Zarma du Niger.* Paris: Anthropos.

Djibo, Hadiza, et al. 1998. *Module de formation. Thème: Islam/population et développement, Niamey.* Projet NER/98/04/01/03 ISLAM/SR/PF.

Donati, Pascale. 2000. "L'absence d'enfant": un choix plus ou moins délibéré dans le parcours d'hommes et de femmes. *Recherches et prévisions* 62: 43–56.

Douglas, Mary. 1986. *How institutions think.* Syracuse: Syracuse University Press.

Echard, Nicole. 1985. Même la viande est vendue avec le sang. De la sexualité des femmes, un exemple. In *L'arraisonnement des femmes: essais en anthropologie des sexes*, ed. Nicole-Claude Mathieu, 37–60. Paris: EHESS.

Echard, Nicole. 1989. *Bori, aspects d'un culte de possession Hausa dans l'Ader et le Kurfey, Niger.* Paris: EHESS.

El Aaddouni, Houda. 2003. Stérilité au féminin: enjeux du corps, enjeux de la mémoire. *Face à face. Des regards sur la santé* (5): 47–53. http://journals.open edition.org/faceaface/418

Elias, Norbert. 1973. *La civilisation des mœurs.* Paris: Calmann-Lévy.

Erny, Pierre. 1988. *Les premiers pas dans la vie de l'enfant d'Afrique noire. Naissance et première enfance.* Paris: L'Harmattan.

Evans-Pritchard, Edward Evan. 1951. *Kinship and marriage among the Nuer.* Oxford: Clarendon Press.

Fainzang, Sylvie. 1991. Sexualité et reproduction chez les Africaines immigrées soninke et toucouleur vivant en ménage polygamique. *Sciences sociales et santé* 9 (4): 89–109.

Fainzang, Sylvie, and Odile Journet. 1989. *La femme de mon mari. Anthropologie du mariage polygamique en Afrique et en France.* Paris: L'Harmattan.

Fainzang, Sylvie, and Odile Journet. 2002. L'institution polygamique comme lieu de construction sociale de la féminité. In *Sexe et genre. De la hiérarchie des sexes*, eds. Marie-Claude Hurtig, Michèle Kail, and Hélène Rouch, 217–225. Paris: CNRS.

FNUAP. 2000. *Rapport annuel du Niger (année 1999).*

FP2030. 2022. Niger FP2030 Indicator summary sheet: 2021–22 annual progress report. Accessed November 10, 2022. http://www.track20.org/Niger

Farge, Arlette. 1997. *Des lieux pour l'histoire.* Paris: Le Seuil.

Fassin, Didier. 1992. *Pouvoir et maladie en Afrique. Anthropologie sociale dans la banlieue de Dakar.* Paris: Presses universitaires de France.

Fassin, Didier, and Dominique Memmi, eds. 2004. *Le gouvernement du corps.* Paris: EHESS.

Febvre, Lucien. 1992. *Combats pour l'histoire.* Paris: Armand Colin.

Fine, Agnès. 2002. Maternité et identité féminine. In *Maternité, affaire privée, affaire publique*, ed. Yvonne Knibiehler, 61–76. Paris: Bayard.

Flandrin, Jean-Louis. 1984. *Familles. Parenté, maison, sexualité dans l'ancienne société.* Paris: Le Seuil.

Foucault, Michel. 1986. *L'histoire de la sexualité I. La volonté de savoir.* Paris: Gallimard.

Fraisse, Geneviève. 1998. *Les femmes et leur histoire.* Paris: Gallimard.

Gélis, Jacques. 1984. *L'arbre et le fruit. La naissance dans l'occident moderne (XVIe et XIXe siècle)*. Paris: Fayard.

Gélis, Jacques, Mireille Laget, and Marie-France Morel. 1978. *Entrer dans la vie. Naissances et enfances dans la France traditionnelle*. Paris: Gallimard/Julliard.

Global Health Observatory. 2019. Maternal mortality ratio (per 100 000 live births): data. Accessed February 17, 2022. https://www.who.int/data/gho/data/indicators/indicator-details/GHO/maternal-mortality-ratio-(per-100-000-live-births).

Gobatto, Isabelle. 1999. *Être médecin au Burkina Faso. Dissection sociologique d'une transplantation professionnelle*. Paris: L'Harmattan.

Gobatto, Isabelle. 2001. Médecins acteurs dans les systèmes de santé. Une étude de cas au Burkina Faso. In *Systèmes et politiques de santé*, ed. Bernard Hours, 137–162. Paris: Karthala.

Goffman, Erving. 1959. *The presentation of self in everyday life*. Garden City, NY: Anchor Books.

Goffman, Erving. 1963. *Stigma: notes on the management of spoiled identity*. Englewood Cliffs, NJ: Prentice Hall.

Goffman, Erving. 1967. *Interaction ritual: essays in face-to-face behavior*. Chicago: Aldine.

Goffman, Erving. 1977. The arrangement between the sexes. *Theory and Society* 4 (3): 301–331.

Goody, Jack. 1969. Adoption in cross-cultural perspective. *Comparative Studies in Society and History* 11 (1): 55–78.

Gruénais, Marc-Eric. 1996. À quoi sert l'hôpital Africain? L'offre des soins à maman Bwale (Brazzaville). *Les annales de la recherche urbaine* 73: 118–128.

Guillaume, Agnès. 2009. L'avortement provoqué en Afrique: un problème mal connu, lourd de conséquences. In *Santé de la reproduction au Nord et au Sud: de la connaissance à l'action: actes de la Chaire Quételet 2004*, ed. Catherine Gourbin, 357–381. Louvain-la-Neuve: Presses universitaires de Louvain.

Hahonou, Eric Komlavi. 2000. *Étude socio-anthropologique des interactions entre usagers et agents de santé: le cas du service des urgences de l'hôpital de Niamey, Niger*. Mémoire de DEA. Marseille: EHESS Marseille.

Hassane, Moulaye, Marthe Doka, and Oumarou Makama Bawa. 2006. *Étude sur les pratiques de l'Islam au Niger. Rapport d'enquête provisoire*. Niamey: DANIDA Bureau de Coopération Danoise.

Haxaire, Claudie. 2003. "Toupaille," kits MST et remèdes du "mal d'enfants" chez les Gouro de Zuénoula (Côte-d'Ivoire). *Anthropologie et sociétés* 27 (2): 77–95.

Héritier, Françoise. 1978. Fécondité et stérilité. La traduction de ces notions dans le champ idéologique au stade pré-scientifique. In *Le fait féminin*, ed. Evelyne Sullerot, 387–396. Paris: Fayard.

Héritier, Françoise. 1984. Stérilité, aridité, sécheresse: quelques invariants de la pensée symbolique. In *Le sens du mal. Anthropologie, histoire et sociologie de la maladie*, eds. Marc Augé and Claudine Herzlich, 123–154. Paris: Éditions des archives contemporaines.

Héritier, Françoise. 1996. *Masculin/féminin: la pensée de la différence*. Paris: Éditions Odile Jacob.

Héritier, Françoise. 2002. *Masculin/féminin II: dissoudre la hiérarchie*. Paris: Éditions Odile Jacob.

Horellou-Lafarge, Chantal. 1982. Une mutation dans les dispositifs du contrôle social: le cas de l'avortement. *Revue française de sociologie* 23 (3): 397–416.

Houel, Annik, and Brigitte Lhomond. 1982. Avortement et morale maternelle 1968–1978. *Revue française de sociologie* 23 (3): 487–502.

Imorou, Abou-Bakari. 2006. Cliniciens versus santé publique: une analyse de la mise en œuvre d'une réforme sanitaire au Bénin. Thèse de doctorat nouveau régime, EHESS Marseille.

Institute National de la Statistique. 2006. *Niger: enquête démographique et de santé et à indicateurs multiples, 2006 (EDSN-MICS III). Rapport de synthèse.* Niamey: Institute National de la Statistique.

Isambert, François-André. 1982. Une sociologie de l'avortement est-elle possible? *Revue française de sociologie* 23 (3): 359–381.

Jaffré, Yannick. 1997. La consultation de gynécologie: une approche globale. *L'enfant en milieu tropical* 231: 2–18.

Jaffré, Yannick. 1999. Pharmacies des villes, pharmacies par terre. *Bulletin de l'APAD* 17: 63–70.

Jaffré, Yannick. 2003a. La description en actes. Que décrit-on, comment, pour qui? In *Pratiques de la description*, eds. Giorgio Blundo and Jean-Pierre Olivier de Sardan, 55–73. Paris: Éditions de l'EHESS.

Jaffré, Yannick. 2003b. La configuration de l'espace moral et psychologique des personnels de santé. In *Une médecine inhospitalière. Les difficiles relations entre soignants et soignés dans cinq capitales d'Afrique de l'Ouest*, eds. Yannick Jaffré and Jean-Pierre Olivier de Sardan, 295–337. Paris: Karthala.

Jaffré, Yannick. 2003c. Le souci de l'autre. Une anthropologie de la santé au risque du terrain. HDR, Université de Provence.

Jaffré, Yannick. 2003d. Le souci de l'autre. Audit, éthique professionnelle et réflexivité des soignants en Guinée. *Autrepart* 28 (4): 95–110.

Jaffré, Yannick, and Jean-Pierre Olivier de Sardan. 2003. Réformer une éthique sous contraintes? In *La médecine inhospitalière. Les difficiles relations entre soignants et soignés dans cinq capitales d'Afrique de l'Ouest*, eds. Yannick Jaffré and Jean-Pierre Olivier de Sardan, 339–358. Paris: Karthala.

Jaffré, Yannick, and Alain Prual. 1993. "Le corps des sages-femmes," entre identité professionnelle et sociale. *Sciences sociales et santé* 11 (2): 63–80.

Journet, Odile. 1985. Les hyper-mères n'ont plus d'enfants. Maternité et ordre social chez les Joola de Basse-Casamance. In *L'arraisonnement des femmes. Essais en anthropologie des sexes*, ed. Nicole Claude Mathieu, 17–36. Paris: Éditions de l'EHESS.

Journet, Odile. 1991. Un rituel de préservation de la descendance, le Kanyaalen Joola. In *Grossesse et petite enfance en Afrique noire et Madagascar*, eds. Suzanne Lallemend, Odile Journet, Elisabeth Ewombe-Moundo, et al., 19–39. Paris: L'Harmattan.

Kang, Alice. 2015. *Bargaining for women's rights: activism in an aspiring Muslim democracy.* Minneapolis: University of Minnesota Press.

Kintz, Danièle. 1987. De l'art peul de l'adultère. *Journal des anthropologues* 29–30 (1): 119–143.

Knibiehler, Yvonne, ed. 2001. *Maternité, affaire privée, affaire publique.* Paris: Bayard.

Konan, Bla Claire, et al. 2005. L'inégale prise en compte de l'autre (exemple de la tuberculose et de la prévention). In *Les professionnels de santé en Afrique de l'Ouest entre savoirs et pratiques*, eds. Laurent Vidal, Abdou Salam Fall, and Dakouri Gadou, 101–136. Paris: L'Harmattan.

Koné, Mariatou. 2000. L'avortement: une pratique contraceptive "sûre" en Côte d'Ivoire? *Réseau anthropologie de la santé en Afrique* 1 (April): 95–104.

Koster, Winny. 2003. *Secret strategies: women and abortion in Yoruba society, Nigeria.* Amsterdam: Aksant.

Lacoste, Michèle. 1993. Langage et interaction: le cas de la consultation médicale. In *Soins et communication. Approche interactionniste des relations de soins*, eds. Jacques Cosnier, Michèle Grosjean, and Michèle Lacoste, 33–61. Lyon: Presses universitaires de Lyon.

Lacoste-Dujardin, Camille. [1985] 1996. *Des mères contre les femmes. Maternité et patriarcat au Maghreb.* Paris: La Découverte.

Laget, Mireille. 1982. *Naissances. L'accouchement avant l'âge clinique.* Paris: Le Seuil.

Lahire, Bernard. 1998. *L'homme pluriel. Les ressorts de l'action.* Paris: Nathan.

Lallemand, Suzanne. 1988a. Un bien qui circule beaucoup. *Autrement* 96: 135–141.

Lallemand, Suzanne. 1988b. Adoption, fosterage et alliance. *Anthropologie et sociétés* 12 (2): 25–40.

Le Breton, David. 2003. *Anthropologie du corps et modernité.* Paris: Presses universitaires de France.

Le Naour, Jean-Yves, and Catherine Valenti. 2003. *Histoire de l'avortement (XIXe–XXe siècle).* Paris: Le Seuil.

Locoh, Thérèse. 1984. *Fécondité et famille en Afrique de l'Ouest. Le Togo méridional contemporain.* Paris: Presses universitaires de France.

Locoh, Thérèse. 1991. Familles dans la crise et politiques de population en Afrique subsaharienne. *Politique Africaine* 44: 78–90.

Locoh, Thérèse, and Jean-Marie Sztalryd. 1995. Le corps assujetti. In *La place des femmes. Les enjeux de l'identité et de l'égalité au regard des sciences sociales*, ed. EPHESIA, 272–279. Paris: La Découverte.

Lutz-Fuchs, Dominique. 1994. *Psychothérapies de femmes Africaines.* Paris: L'Harmattan.

Maisonneuve, Jean. 1993. *Les sentiments.* Paris: Presses universitaires de France.

Masquelier, Adeline. 2001. *Prayer has spoiled everything: possession, power, and identity in an Islamic town of Niger.* Durham, NC: Duke University Press.

Massard, Josiane. 1988. L'adoption ou la quasi-parentalité/parenté fictive ou partielle. *Anthropologie et sociétés* 12 (1): 41–62.

Mathieu, Nicole-Claude, ed. 1985. *L'arraisonnement des femmes. Essais en anthropologie des sexes.* Paris: Éditions de l'EHESS.

Maulet, Nathalie, Mahamoudou Keita, and Jean Macq. 2013. Medico-social pathways of obstetric fistula patients in Mali and Niger: an 18-month cohort follow-up. *Tropical Medicine & International Health* 18 (5): 524–533.

Mauss, Marcel. 1954. *The gift: forms and functions of exchange in archaic societies.* London: Cohen & West.

McLaren, Angus. 1990. *A history of contraception: from antiquity to the present day.* Oxford: Basil Blackwell.

Meillassoux, Claude. 1975. *Femmes, greniers et capitaux.* Paris: François Maspero.

Meyer, Larissa, Charles Ascher-Walsh, Rachael Norman, et al. 2007. Commonalities among women who experienced vesicovaginal fistulae as a result of obstetric trauma in Niger: results from a survey given at the National Hospital Fistula Center, Niamey, Niger. *American Journal of Obstetrics and Gynecology* 197 (1): 90.e1–90.e4.

Mgalla, Zaida, and Jan Ties Boerma. 2002. The discourse on infertility in Tanzania. In *Women and infertility in sub-Saharan African: a multidisciplinary perspective*, eds. Jan Ties Boerma and Zaida Mgalla, 189–200. Amsterdam: Kit Publishers.

Monfouga-Nicolas, Jacqueline. 1972. *Ambivalence et culte de possession.* Paris: Anthropos.

Mottin Sylla, Marie-Hélène. 1997. Le libre choix en matière de sexualité et de fécondité. In *Femmes et Africaines. Un double combat,* 139–154. Dakar: ENDA.

Moumouni, Adamou. 2000. Conceptions et pratiques de l'avortement en pays Songhy-Zarma. *Réseau anthropologie de la santé en Afrique* 1 (April): 104–109.

Moussa, Hadiza. 2003. Niamey: le complexe sanitaire de Boukoki. In *Une médecine inhospitalière. Les difficiles relations entre soignants et soignés dans cinq capitales de l'Afrique de l'Ouest,* eds. Yannick Jaffré and Jean-Pierre Olivier de Sardan, 361–385. Paris: Karthala.

Moussa, Hadiza. 2004a. Devoir de soigner et droit d'exercer la violence: ethnographie des consultations de planification familiale à Niamey/Niger. *Bulletin de l'APAD* 25 (June): 49–67.

Moussa, Hadiza. 2004b. La pratique de la planification familiale en milieu rural: cas du district sanitaire de Kollo. *Études et travaux du LASDEL* 23: 1–53.

Moussa Abdallah, Hadiza. 2001. La pharmacie par terre: une alternative à l'échec de la politique pharmaceutique nationale? Étude de cas dans la commune Niamey III. Mémoire de maîtrise de sociologie, Université de Ouagadougou.

Moussa Abdallah, Hadiza. 2002. Micro-analyse des interactions autour des consultations de planification familiale dans les centres des soins de Niamey. DEA en sciences sociales, EHESS Marseille.

Nasr, Seyyed Hossein. 2000. *Ideals and reality of Islam.* Chicago: ABC International Group.

Olivier de Sardan, Jean-Pierre. 1982. *Concepts et conceptions Songhay-Zarma.* Paris: Nubia.

Olivier de Sardan, Jean-Pierre. 1984. *Les sociétés Songhay-Zarma (Mali-Niger). Chefs, guérriers, esclaves, paysans.* Paris: Karthala.

Olivier de Sardan, Jean-Pierre. 1995. La politique du terrain. Sur la production des données en anthropologie. *Enquête, anthropologie, histoire, sociologie* 1: 71–109.

Olivier de Sardan, Jean-Pierre. 1999a. Introduction. In *La construction sociale des maladies. Les entités nosologiques populaires en Afrique de l'Ouest,* eds. Yannick Jaffré and Jean-Pierre Olivier de Sardan, 7–12. Paris: Presses universitaires de France.

Olivier de Sardan, Jean-Pierre. 1999b. Les entités nosologiques populaires internes: quelques logiques représentationnelles. In *La construction sociale des maladies. Les entités nosologiques populaires en Afrique de l'Ouest,* eds. Yannick Jaffré and Jean-Pierre Olivier de Sardan, 71–87. Paris: Presses universitaires de France.

Olivier de Sardan, Jean-Pierre. 2000. Le "je" méthodologique. Implication et explicitation dans l'enquête de terrain. *Revue française de sociologie* 41 (3): 417–445.

Olivier de Sardan, Jean-Pierre. 2001a. Populisme méthodologique et populisme idéologique. In *Le goût de l'enquête,* ed. Jean-Louis Fabiani, 195–246. Paris: L'Harmattan.

Olivier de Sardan, Jean-Pierre. 2001b. La sage-femme et le douanier. Cultures professionnelles locales et culture bureaucratique privatisée en Afrique de l'Ouest. *Autrepart* 20 (4): 61–73.

Omondi-Odhiambo. 1997. Men's participation in family planning decisions in Kenya. *Population Studies* 51 (1): 29–40.

Omran, Abdel-Rahim. 1992. *Family planning in the legacy of Islam.* London: Routledge.

Ouattara, Fatoumata. 1999. Savoir-vivre et honte chez les Senoufo nanerge (Burkina Faso). Thèse de doctorat nouveau régime, EHESS Marseille.

Ouattara, Fatoumata. 2004. Une étrange familiarité. Les exigences de l'anthropologie "chez soi." *Cahiers d'études Africaines* 175: 635–657.

Pasian, Michela. 2010. *Anthropologie du rituel de possession Bori en milieu Hawsa au Niger.* Paris: L'Harmattan.

Paulme, Denise. 1986. *La mère dévorante. Essai sur la morphologie des contes africains.* Paris: Gallimard.

Pilon, Marc, and Agnès Guillaume. 2000. *Maîtrise de la fécondité et planification familiale au Sud.* Paris: IRD Éditions.

Pourchez, Laurence. 2002. *Grossesse, naissance et petite enfance en société créole (Île de la Réunion).* Paris: Karthala and CRDP Réunion.

Rasmussen, Susan J. 2012. Spirit possession in Africa. In *The Wiley-Blackwell companion to African religions*, ed. Elias Kifon Bongma, 184–97. Hoboken, NJ: John Wiley & Sons.

Ravololomanga, Bodo. 1992. *Être femme et mère à Madagascar.* Paris: L'Harmattan.

Renne, Elisha P. 1997. The meaning of contraceptive choice constraint for Hausa women in a northern Nigerian town. *Anthropology and medicine* 4 (2): 159–175.

Retel-Laurentin, Anne. 1974. *Infécondité en Afrique Noire. Maladies et conséquences sociales.* Paris: Éditions Masson et Cie.

Revel, Jacques. 1996. *Jeux d'échelle. La micro-analyse à l'expérience.* Paris: Gallimard/ Le Seuil.

Rich, Adrienne. 1995. *Of woman born: motherhood as experience and institution.* New York: W. W. Norton & Co.

Rivière, Claude. 1990. *Union et procréation en Afrique. Rites de la vie chez les Evé du Togo.* Paris: L'Harmattan.

Ryckmans, Hélène. 1997. Les associations féminines en Afrique: une décennie d'ajustement après la décennie de la femme. In *Face aux changements, les femmes du Sud*, ed. Jeanne Bissiliat, 195–219. Paris: L'Harmattan.

Sala-Diakanda, Francis, and S. Kassegne. 2001. Les idéaux en matière de fécondité: une analyse au niveau du couple. Paper presented at the Colloque international Genre, population et développement en Afrique, Abidjan 16– 21 July.

Santiago-Delefosse, Marie. 1995. *Fécondation in vitro. Demande d'enfant et pratiques médicales.* Paris: Anthropos.

Sartre, Jean Paul. [1943] 1983. *Being and nothingness.* Hazel E. Barnes (trans.). New York: Pocket Books.

Scott, James. 1985. *Weapons of the weak: everyday forms of peasant resistance.* London: Yale University Press.

Shorter, Edward. 1984. Les désordres "hystériques" sont-ils psychosomatiques? *Cahiers internationaux de sociologie* 76: 201–224.

Sindzingre, Nicole. 1984. L'explication de l'infortune chez les Senufo. In *Le sens du mal. Anthropologie, histoire et sociologie de la maladie*, eds. Marc Augé and Cladine Herzlich, 93–122. Paris: Éditions des archives contemporaines.

Smith, Mary F. 1954. *Baba of Karo: a woman of the Muslim Hausa.* London: Faber and Faber.

Souley, Aboubacar. 2003. Un environnement inhospitalier. In *Une médecine inhospitalière. Les difficiles relations entre soignants et soignés dans cinq capitales d'Afrique de l'Ouest*, eds. Yannick Jaffré and Jean-Pierre Olivier de Sardan, 105– 155. Paris: Karthala.

Sounaye, Abdoulaye. 2021. The Salafi revolution in West Africa. *Politique africaine* 161–162 (1–2): 403–425.

Sounaye, Abdoulaye, Aïssa Diarra, and Issa Younoussi. 2017. Genre et population: étude socio-anthropologique sur les déterminants des politiques de population au Niger. *Études et travaux du LASDEL* 123: 1–89.

Sow, Fatou, and Codou Bop. 2004. *Notre corps, notre santé. La santé et la sexualité des femmes en Afrique subsaharienne*. Paris: L'Harmattan.

Stoller, Paul. 1995. *Embodying colonial memories: spirit possession, power, and the Hauka in West Africa*. New York: Routledge.

Stork, Hélène. 1999. *Introduction à la psychologie anthropologique*. Paris: Armand Colin.

Tabet, Paola. 1998. *La construction sociale de l'inégalité des sexes*. Paris: L'Harmattan.

Tchak, Sami. 1999. *La sexualité féminine en Afrique. Domination masculine et libération féminine*. Paris: L'Harmattan.

Thiriat, Marie-Paule. 1998. *Faire et défaire les liens du mariage. Evolution des pratiques matrimoniales au Togo*. Les études du CEPED 16. Paris: Centre français sur la population et le développement.

Tichit, Christine. 2009. Les conséquences sociales de la stérilité au Cameroun. In *Santé de la reproduction au Nord et au Sud: de la connaissance à l'action: actes de la Chaire Quételet 2004*, ed. Catherine Gourbin, 237–276. Louvain-la-Neuve: Presses universitaires de Louvain.

Tiékoura, Ouassa. 1997. Forme communautaire et forme individuelle de la prostitution à Niamey. In *L'Afrique des individus: Itinéraires citadins dans l'Afrique contemporaine (Abidjan, Bamako, Dakar, Niamey)*, eds. Alain Marie, Robert Vuarin, François Leimdorfer, et al., 329–365. Paris: Karthala.

UNAIDS. 2020. Niger 2020 country factsheet. Accessed February 17, 2022. https://www.unaids.org/en/regionscountries/countries/niger

United Nations Inter-agency Group for Child Mortality Estimation. 2021. Niger. Accessed June 16, 2021. https://childmortality.org/data/Niger.

United Nations Population Fund. 2000. *Rapport annuel du Niger (année 1999), August*.

United Nations Population Fund. 2022. World population dashboard: Niger. Accessed February 17, 2022. https://www.unfpa.org/data/world-population/NE.

Wade, Kodou. 2001. Comportements relationnels et fécondité des mères à Ouakam dans l'agglomération dakaroise (Sénégal). Thèse de doctorat nouveau régime, EHESS Paris.

Zempléni, András. 1985. La "maladie" et ses "causes": introduction. *L'ethnographie* 96–97 (2–3): 13–44.

INDEX

For the benefit of digital users, indexed terms that span two pages (e.g., 52–53) may, on occasion, appear on only one of those pages.

Tables and figures are indicated by *t* and *f* following the page number

condoms, contraception with, 129–30, 165

confiage. See fostering

confidentiality, concerns in biomedical
settings over, 137–39

conjugal abstinence, 151–52, 156–
57, 184–85

conjugal debt, 210

normative marriage in Niger and, 8–9

consent of patients, biomedical decision-
making and omission of, 123–26

contraception
abortion and, 188–89, 192–93
barriers for single women to, 190–91
barrier methods, 129n.8
belts for, 159–64
in biomedical setting, 129–31, 135–37,
139–43, 211–12
conjugal transactions over, 3, 173–77
difficulties with biomedical
regimens, 118
economic motivations for, 148–49
family recipes for, 157–58
HIV/AIDS and, 171–72
infertility linked to, 119
informal networks for knowledge and
practices of, 155–59
itinerant pharmacists and, 164–66
management in Niger of, 1
marital strategies and practice
and, 183–85
natural practices for, 155–57
Nigerien women's experiences with, 22
polygamy and use of, 183–85
popular therapeutic specialists
in, 159–64
prevalence rate in Niger, 10–11
religious debates over, 169–72
reproductive health and, 1–2
rhythm method and, 157
self-medication and do-it-yourself
methods, 158–59
side effects, 131–32
social norms concerning, 5–6, 148–
55, 167–69
stigmatization in Niger of, xiv
subversion of power through, 180–82
traditional and magico-religious
techniques, 147
in West Africa, xi

Convention on the Elimination of All
Forms of Discrimination Against
Women, 170–71

Cooper, Barbara, xiv

Corbin, Alain, 96

Cosnier, Jacques, 133

Côte d'Ivoire, infertility and witchcraft in, 33

Countless Blessings (Cooper), xviii

cousins, marriage between, 73

Cox, Susan, xviii

curative baths, infertility management
and, 59

death, sterility as symbolic death, 32, 84, 104

debt of life, guilt of childless women
concerning, 106–8

de Gaulejac, Vincent, 110

demography
of Niger, 10–12
social contract and, 196

denudation, as infertility treatment, 34

Department of Reproductive Health
(Direction de la Santé de la
Reproduction [DSR]) (Niger), 9

Depo-Provera, 130

despair, of infertile women, 111–13

Deutsch, Hélène, 155

Diarra, Aissa, 188n.1

dilation and curettage, 204–6

Diouldé, Fatima, 15

divine grace, amenorrhea linked to, 39–40

divorce
bridewealth and, 35n.4
infertility and, 70
male infertility and, 26, 27–28, 38
polygamy as protection from, 61–64
of sterile women, 34–35

doctors. *See* biomedical contraception;
biomedical fertility management

do-it-yourself contraceptive methods, 158–59

double bind theory, 208n.2

Douglas, Mary, 168

Duchesne, Veronique, xiii

Durkheim, Émile, 108

Echard, Nicole, xvi, 1–2

École des Hautes Études en Sciences
Sociales (EHESS), xv–xvi, xviii

École des Maris, family planning education
in, 175n.7

economic conditions
contraception and, 148–49
fostering as response to, 68–69
itinerant pharmaceutical vendors
and, 164–66

education, for Nigerien women and girls, 190–91, 209
ego, pejoration of, in infertile women, 111
El Aaddouni, Houda, 29
emotions
    anthropology of, 96–97
    infertility management and, 213–14
    obstacles to research on, 97–98
empathy, absence in biomedical settings of, 132–39
endo-ethnology
    fertility research, 12–18
    interview setting in, 16–17, 16*t*
    limitations of, 19–20
    semiology as element of, 20–21
    summary of observations, 18, 18*t*
entourage
    contraceptive subversion and use of, 181, 191
    of married women, 196
Entre absence et refus d'enfant:
    Socioanthropologie de la gestion de la
    fécondité féminine à Niamey, Niger
    (2012) (Moussa), xviii
Erny, Pierre, 32
Evans-Pritchard, Hugh, 43
evil eye, infertility and, 46–47
excision, 99, 210
exclusion of childless women
    by family members, 102–4
    infertility and forms of, 100–5
    from marital lineage, 101–2
    in marriage, 100
    self-exclusion, 104–5
    social marginalization, 104
extended family. *See* family structure
extra-marital pregnancy, 28
    abortion and, 43, 190–91
    male infertility and, 74
extra-marital sex, infertility linked to, 42–43, 56

face, shame of childlessness and loss of, 108–9
Fainzang, Sylvie, xvi, 151–52, 185
family code (Niger), 169–70
family planning in Niger, xii–xiii. *See also* birth spacing; contraception
family structure
    biomedical management of fertility and, 126–27

contraceptive use and monitoring in, 6, 175–76
ethnographic research and, 15
exclusion within, 102–4
fertility management and role of, 2–3, 15, 17, 128–29
infertility and exclusion from, 63
intergenerational transmission and continuity of, 84–85
marginalization by in-laws, 101–2
marital relationships within, 176–77
older woman as "mother of newborn" in, 156–57
polygamy and, 64
transactions over contraception and, 173–77
Farge, Arlette, 96
Fassin, Didier, 164
fasting, infertility treatment and, 59
fault, childlessness and feelings of, 107
fear, subfertility and, 91–92
Febvre, Lucien, 96
Feldman-Savelsberg, Pamela, xvi
femininity
    amenorrhea as abnormality of, 38–40
    motherhood tied to, 3, 17, 34, 38–40
    semiology concerning, 20–21
    symbolic representations of fertility linked to, 30–32
fertility. *See also* contraception
    bodily impediments to conception, 38–41
    components of, 20
    ethnographic research on, 12–18, 14*f*
    family structure and, 2–3, 15, 17, 128–29
    fostering as aid to, 66
    infertility dialectic with, 30
    methodological challenges of research on, 19–20
    occult practices and thwarting of, 44–48
    regulation in Africa of, 1–2
    revenue-driven management protocols for, 121–23
    sexuality and, 4–5
    social norms in Niger about, 2–3, 4, 5–6, 148–55
    stigmatization of closely-spaced pregnancies, 152–55
    study sites for research on, 13–15
    suspended fertility, sleeping embryo and, 37–38, 48–49

symbolic representations of, 30–32
  as women's responsibility, 9–10, 28–30
fertility compression, xii–xiii
fertility rates
  in Niger, xxv, 10–12, 10f
fertility reduction, xii–xiii
fistulas, postpartum, 127
food, male impotence linked, 55
food insecurity, infant and maternal
  mortality in Niger and, 11–12
forced marriage, 193
force of blood, 44
force of milk, 44
fostering
  as fertility aid, 66
  by grandparents, 103–4
  infertility management and, 64–69
  as life work, 69
  postponement of, 69
  stigmatization of, 67–68
Foucault, Michel, 5
foyandi social groups, 16–17
France
  abortion in, 196, 198
  frequent pregnancy and women's well-
    being in, 155
  women's responsibility for
    infertility in, 29

Gaudio, Rudy, xvii
Gélis, Jacques, xv–xvi, 204
gender dynamics
  fertility management and, 20
  gender hierarchies and, 1–2
  infertility and, 34
  male impotence and, 54
  marriage and sexuality and, xvi
  sexual control and, 4–5
  spirit possession and, xvii
gender quota system, 170–71
genital cutting. *See* circumcision;
    excision
Ghana, infertility treatment rituals in, 60
The Gift (Mauss), 208
global health, contraception and, 167
Gobatto, Isabelle, 140–41
Goffman, Erving, xvi, 20, 108, 110,
    133, 196
grand multipara women, 140n.12
grandparents, role in childbearing
    of, 103–4
Guillaume, Agnès, 191

guilt
  childlessness and feelings of, 25–28, 32–
    33, 105–10, 214
  debt of life obligation and, 106–8
  pre-marital sex linked to infertility
    and, 41–42
gyneco-obstetric surgery, 120

haawi. See shame
Hausa culture, reproductive health and, xvii
hawari contraceptive practice, 160–64
health workers. *See* biomedical
    contraception; biomedical infertility
    management
herbal medicines
  abortion using, 201–2
  do-it-yourself contraceptive methods
    and, 158–59
  infertility treatment and, 59–60
  traditional contraceptive methods and,
    53–56, 164
Héritier, Françoise, xvi, 29, 30–31, 40–41,
    50–51, 72, 95
Hertrich, Véronique, xvi
heteronormativity, reproductive health
    research and, xvii–xviii
*A History of Contraception: From Antiquity to
    the Present Day* (McLaren), 6
HIV/AIDS, 53, 129
  contraception policy and, 171–72
  in Niger, 11–12
  reproductive health and, 1–2
holy water, infertility treatments
    with, 58–59
hope, of infertile women, 111–13
Horbst, Viola, xiii–xiv
Horellou-Lafarge, Chantal, 196
hospitals/health clinics. *See* biomedical
    contraception; biomedical infertility
    management
Houel, Annik, 192
humiliation, of adultery, 72
humor, stigmatization of sterility with, 35
husbands
  biomedical management of fertility
    and, 126–27
  fertility research and, 17
  reluctance about sterility treatment
    in, 26–28
hysterectomy, 123
hysterography, 119
hysterosalpingography, 119–20

immortality, fertility linked to, 32–33
Imorou, Abou-Bakari, 206
impotence
    male infertility and, 26–28, 38
    prevention of, 54–55
incest, infertility and, 43–44, 53–54
infanticide, 195–96
infant mortality
    close pregnancies linked to, 11, 152–55
    as forgotten fertility, case studies
        of, 86–89
    rate in Niger, 11
Infécondité en afrique noire
        (Retel-Laurentin), xiii
infertile sexuality, xxvii–xxviii, 1, 7, 207
    abortion as a form of, 187
infertility
    abortion disguised as, 193–95
    adultery linked to, 42–43, 70–74
    in Africa, research on, xii–xiv
    anthropology of emotions and, 96–97,
        213–14
    biomedical decision-making process
        for, 123–26
    biomedical procedures and costs
        for, 118–23
    black magic and, 44, 45–46
    blood incompatibility linked to, 37–
        38, 40–41
    definitions of, xii–xiii, xix
    divorce and remarriage as response to, 70
    fostering as management of, 64–
        69, 79–81
    hardships for infertile women, 77–79
    incestuous sexuality and, 43–44
    intergenerational transmission, 84–85
    in males, 26–28, 54–55
    management of, 1, 52–53, 61–74
    marabouts and management of, 57–
        59, 81
    marginalization by family, 102–4
    marital difficulties and, 80
    meaning and causation for, 37–38
    medical management of, 53, 74–75, 81
    miscarriages and, 79–81
    Nigerien social construction of, 21–22
    patients' lack of knowledge about, 124
    polygamy as management of,
        61–64, 81–85
    prevention of, 53–56
    sexuality and, xxvii–xxviii, 92–95
    social and emotional experiences with, xiii

social control of, 5–6
as social death, 32–33
social typology of, 76
spirit possession and, 47–48
stigmatization of, xvi
traditional healers and management
    of, 59–60
transgenerational misalignment
    and, 49–50
treatment of, 56–60
in West Africa, xi
witchcraft and, 33–34
infidelity. *See* adultery
informal networks of fertility
    practices, 2
inheritance
    fostering and, 65
    polygamy and, 184
    wealth transference and, 84–85
Inhorn, Marcia, xiii
intergenerational transmission, family
    continuity and, 84
interview setting, ethnographic research
    and, 16–17
intrauterine device (IUD), 130, 132, 135, 142
involuntary infertility, social control of, 6
Isambert, François-André, 191, 196
Islam in Niger
    abortion and, 197–98
    adoption in, 65
    amenorrhea linked to divine grace
        in, 39–40
    contraception and, 169–72
    fundamentalism of, xxvii
    infertility prevention and, 42–43, 56
    infertility treatment in, 57–59
    marital sex and, 8, 156, 157
    polygamy and, 185
    semiology concerning sexuality in, 20–21
    sleeping embryo myth and, 48–49

Jaffré, Yannick, 63, 96, 97–98, 117,
    134, 164
Jamiyat Nassaratul Dine
    association, 170n.2
jealousy
    fertility reignited through, 62–63
    polygamy and, xxvii
    witchcraft and infertility and, 44, 46–47
Johnson-Hanks, Jennifer, xvi
Joola people (Casamance), 73
Journet, Odile, 73, 102, 183

microstrategies of women
contraceptive subversion and, 180–82
manipulation of social norms through,
6, 177–80
silent resistance and, 214–15
mifepristone (RU-486), 204–5
milk. *See* bad milk; breastfeeding
miscarriage
abortion disguised as, 192, 195–96
semiology surrounding, 198–99
women's experiences with, 79–81
misoprostol, 204–5
mobile phones, popular healers use of, 58
modesty, concerns in biomedical settings
over, 137–39
monogamous households, women's sexual
obligations in, 8
moonlight, female infertility and, 56
Mossi culture, 31–32, 33–34, 49–50
motherhood
as competitive strategy in polygamous
marriage, 183–85
contradictory norms about, 208
femininity linked to, 3, 17, 34
fostering as aid to, 66
infant mortality as negation of, 88–89
overvaluation of, 107
primacy of, 61–62
professional success as replacement
for, 93–95
social role of, 57
subfertility and, 92
subfertility as failure of, 91
symbolic representations of fertility
linked to, 30–32
women's social existence linked to, 3, 17
Mottin Sylla, Marie Hélène, 210
Moussa, Hadiza
death of, xviii
reproductive health research by, xi
theoretical orientations and absences in
work of, xv–xviii
translation of work, xviii–xx

naming
infertility and loss of, 84
in weddings and funeral
announcements, 91n.14
National Center for Reproductive Health
(Centre National de la Santé de la
Reproduction), 13, 130
neem leaf, 159, 201

Niamey, Niger
fertility and infertility concepts in, 25
methodological challenges of fertility
research in, 19–20
Moussa's research in, xvii
population of, 12
private radio stations in, 57–58
Niger
abortion in, xiv–xv, 202
biomedical settings in, 117–18
childbirth in, xiv
ethnographic research on fertility in,
12–18, 14f
fertility rate in, xxv
fostering in, 65–69
infertility rates in, xii–xiii
Islamic fundamentalism in, 169–70
male domination in, xxvii
maternal mortality rate in, xxv
media age of population in, 12
population demographics in, 10–12, 10f
population growth in, xii
reproductive health in, 9–10
sexuality in, 7–9
Nigeria
abortion in, 206
contraceptive use in, 175
divorce and infertility in, 70
infertility linked to pre-marital sex
in, 41–42
Nigerien Association of Muslim
Women, 170n.2
non-governmental organizations (NGOs),
reproductive health in Niger
and, 9–10
nurses. *See* biomedical contraception;
biomedical infertility management
nursing. *See* breastfeeding

observational research, summary of,
18, 18t
occult practices, thwarting of fertility
and, 44–48
Ogino-Knaus contraceptive method, 157
Olivier de Sardan, Jean-Pierre, xviii, xx, 45,
49, 117, 133
oral contraceptives, 130–31, 165
Ouattara, Fatoumata, 105–6
oxytocin, 122, 205

paternity
ambiguity in Niger of, 26–28

male infertility and, 38
  as survival, 32
Paulme, Denise, 33
persecution, of sterile women, 34–35
pharmaceuticals, itinerant vendors of, 15,
  17, 52, 131, 164–66, 181–82
  abortion and, 202–4
placenta
  of animals, traditional medicine and, 59
  burial of, 56
pleasure, women's obligations
  concerning, 8
polio vaccination, Islamic protests
  against, 169
polygamy
  agency of women in, 179–80, 182
  anterior and posterior integration
    in, 61–62
  blood incompatibility of partners
    and, 40–41
  childbearing as competitive strategy
    in, 183–85
  conjugal guerrilla tactics and, 8
  infertility management through, 61–64,
    65, 74, 81–85
  in Niger, xxvii
  paternity recognition and, 28
popular medicine. See also traditional
    healers
  contraceptives and, 131, 159–64
  fertility regulation through, 212–13
  infertility management and, 52–53,
    57, 74–75
population control, xii
population growth and demographics, xii,
  10–12, 10f
posterior integration, in polygamy, 61–62
postpartum abstinence, 151–52, 156–
  57, 184–85
posture, infertility treatments with, 59
potassium permanganate, as
  abortifacient, 201
Pourchez, Laurence, 29, 65, 113
power
  biomedical decision making and role of,
    123–26, 211–12
  in biomedical settings, 117–18
  contraception and subversion of,
    180–82
  reproductive capacity and, 4–5
pragmatic contexts, fertility management
  and, xxv, 212

pregnancy. See also birth spacing
  bad milk for unweaned babies linked
    to, 150–52
  postpartum weight gain and, 156–57
  protection rites for, 56
  stigmatization of closely-spaced
    pregnancies, 152–55
pre-marital pregnancy
  abortion and, 190–91
  acceptance of, 41–42
  avoidance in Niger of, 7–8
pre-marital sex
  consequences in Niger of, 7
  infertility linked to, 41–42
prenatal care, absence in Niger of, 11–12
privacy, concerns in biomedical settings
  over, 137–39
private radio stations, 57–58
procreation
  disjunction with pleasure and, 210
  social promotion of, 4, 6
  subfertility and, 90
  value systems based on, 104
professional success, as replacement for
  children, 93–95
prolactin, contraception and, 155
pro-natalism
  claims to women's bodies and, 211
  contradictory reproductive health
    standards and, 208–9
  economic motivations for contraception
    vs., 148, 153
  fertility control and, 211
  infant mortality and, 11, 154
  motherhood status and, xxvi
  repeated pregnancies and, 90
  social norms and influence of,
    167–69
  stigmatization of contraception and,
    xiv, 147
prostitution in Niamey, desire for
    motherhood linked to, 42
psychological disturbance
  pregnancy and, 68
  shame and, 110
  sterility and, 36n.7, 104–5, 107, 118,
    128–29, 155, 213–14
  subfertility and, 91–92

Ravololomanga, Bodo, 30–31, 32, 33–
  34, 105
remarriage, infertility and, 70

reproductive health
  biological and social dimensions of, 3–5
  close pregnancies as threat to, 149–
    50, 152–55
  commercialization of care, 121
  contradictory standards in, 208–9
  globalization of, 9–10
  government medical facilities and, xix
  intergenerational transmission
    and, 77–85
  in Niger, 9–10
  power of, 4–5
  structural contexts of data on,
    xxv–xxvi
  study sites for research on, 13–15
  in West Africa, xi
  women's identity linked to, 50–51
Reproductive Health and the Advancement
  of Women in Islam (Santé de la
  Reproduction et Promotion de la
  Femme en Islam) project, 171–72
repudiation, polygamy as protection
  from, 61–64
Retel-Laurentin, Anne, xiii
Réunion, 65
Revel, Jacques, 96
Rich, Adrienne, 91
rumors
  contraception techniques and, 131–
    32, 202
  polygamy and, 185

sacrifices, fertility prevention and, 53
Salafism, 57
  in Niger, xxvii
salpingectomy, 119–20, 123
Santiago-Delafosse, Marie, 85, 121
Sargent, Carolyn, 3
Sassens, Saskia, xvi
Sasser, Jade, xii–xiii
schoolgirls. See also education
  abortion association with, 190–91
secondary infertility, 32, 54, 56
self-acceptance, childlessness and loss
  of, 111
self-confidence, childlessness and loss
  of, 111
self-exclusion, by childless
  women, 104–5
self-medication contraceptives, 158–59
self-ownership, multiple claims to women's
  bodies and, 210–11

semiology
  around abortion, 198–99
  in endo-ethnographic research, 20–21
  of infertility, xvi
  of sterility, 34–37
  of witchcraft, 45
Senegal, abortion care in, xv
sensibilités. See emotions
sexual abstinence during breastfeeding,
  151–52, 156–57, 184–85
sexuality. See also infertile sexuality
  agency of women in relation to, 177–80
  disjunction with procreation
    and, 210
  fertility and, 4–5, 34
  gender dynamics in Niger for, xvi
  normative marriage and, 7–9
  polygamy and, 179–80
  semiology concerning, 20–21
  silence in Niger about, 7–8, 19–20
  social norms concerning, 4, 55–56
  stigmatization of, 1
  symbolic representations of fertility
    linked to, 30–32
sexually transmitted diseases/infections
  (STDs/STIs), 53, 126
  in Niger, 11–12
sexual transgression, infertility linked to,
  37–38, 41–44
shame
  childlessness and feelings of, 105–10
  epistemological approach to, 108–9
  haawi in Songhai-Zarma culture
    as, 109–10
  modesty and confidentiality concerns
    and, 117–18
  over abortion, 191
  over pregnancy, 151
  psychology of, 110
  transgenerational conflict and, 50
sheep's liver, infertility treatments
  with, 58–59
simulated sexual acts, as infertility
  treatment, 34
Sindzingre, Nicole, 37
single women
  exclusion from contraception of, 190–91
  stigmatization of, 63–64
skin color, infidelity linked to, 73
sleeping child myth
  contraception and, 163
  infertility and, 37–38, 48–49

Union for the Promotion of Nigerien
    Women, 169–70
Union of Muslim Women in Niger, 170n.2
United Nations Children's Fund
    (UNICEF), 9
United Nations Population Fund (UNFPA),
    9, 171–72

Valenti, Catherine, 153
venereal disease, 119
virginity
    obligation in Niger of, 7
    semiology concerning, 21
virility. *See* masculinity

water spirits, 59
wealth
    bridewealth, 35n.4
    children as, 3, 25, 91
    reproduction and, 84–85
weaning, pregnancy during, 150–52
West Africa, social perceptions of
    sterility in, 37
Western culture
    perceptions of Niger's population growth
    in, xii

stigmatization of sterility based on
    adoption of, 36
witchcraft. *See also* black magic
    infertility and, 33–34, 37–38, 45
withdrawal (coitus interruptus, *al asl*) as
    contraceptive method, 157, 171
womanhood
    infertility and, 92–95
women
    agency in Niger of, 177–80
    fertility responsibilities of, 9–10, 28–30
    guilt for infertility in, 25–28
    infertility prevention for, 55–56
    Islamic fundamentalism in Niger and
        role of, 169–72
    multiple claims to bodies of,
        210–11
worked rooster contraceptive method, 160
written water, as contraceptive, 160

Younoussi, Issa, 188n.1

Zambia, abortion in, xiv–xv
Zangaou, Moussa, xviii
Zarma culture, reproductive health and,
    xvii